I am delighted to present the latest edition of "We Have Kidney Cancer," a resource for patients, families and caregivers.

A diagnosis of kidney cancer can be a significant challenge and feel overwhelming. This book serves as a basic guide to kidney cancer, helping explain the fundamentals of the disease and its treatment, and providing information about resources that can help those dealing with the challenges of a kidney cancer diagnosis.

In recent years a variety of new therapies have been approved by the FDA for the treatment of kidney cancer, and others are in development. Innovative research by dedicated scientists, doctors and nurses is making it possible to treat kidney cancer in new ways – and that offers renewed hope in the lives of kidney cancer patients.

When I began my work as a surgeon, the treatment options for patients were quite limited. Today, there are many promising options, and the updated and expanded content in this edition of "We Have Kidney Cancer" reflects the progress we have made. I am honored to provide the Foreword for this new edition.

As you read, keep in mind that a kidney cancer survivor – one who has already experienced what you and your family are going through – is a good source of information and inspiration. We encourage you to read the testimonials of survivors contained in this book. Their words can help. My experience in working with kidney cancer patients is that they can have a good quality of life, despite a cancer diagnosis.

While this book is comprehensive and complete, you can find other useful resources at our website, www.kidneycancer.com, which is the kidney cancer community's most trusted source of information.

Christopher Wood, MD
Board Chair
Kidney Cancer Association

Acknowledgements

We gratefully acknowledge the commitment of time and the thoughtful input of the kidney cancer patients who reviewed this book and offered their advice to help other patients. Your efforts are deeply appreciated.

We also wish to thank the following individuals who reviewed and commented on this book:

Editorial Directors

Nancy Moldawer, RN, MSN
Cedars-Sinai Medical Center

Laura Wood, RN, MSN, OCN
Cleveland Clinic Taussig Cancer Institute

The Nurse Advisory Board of the Kidney Cancer Association

Nancy Ainslie, RN, BSN
M.D. Anderson Cancer Center (retired)

Laurie Appleby, MS, APRN, BC
Dana-Farber Cancer Institute

Patricia A Creel, RN, BSN,OCN,CCRP
Duke University Medical Center

Patty Fischer, RN, MSN,OCN
Memorial Sloan-Kettering Cancer Center

Jan Jackson, RN
M.D. Anderson Cancer Center

Nancy Moldawer, RN, MSN, Co-Chair
Cedars-Sinai Medical Center

Lynda Pyle, SRN, BSc in Oncology, FETC
The Royal Marsden Hospital, London

Jon Smith, RN, BSN
Seattle Cancer Care Alliance

Sherry Soeder, RN, MSN, CNP
Cleveland Clinic Taussig Cancer Institute/Radiation

Laura Wood, RN, MSN, OCN, Co-Chair
Cleveland Clinic Taussig Cancer Institute

Board of Directors of the Kidney Cancer Association

Paula E. Bowen
Retired College Administrator, New York

Ronald M. Bukowski, MD
Bukowski Consulting, LLC
Cleveland Clinic Taussig Cancer Institute
Cleveland, OH

Noah Buntman
Operations Program Manager, Apple, California

Craig DePriester
DaVita HealthCare Partners, California

James Larkin,Ph.D.
Consultant Medical Oncologist, Royal Marsden Hospital, London and Sutton

Michael B. Lawing
Cancer Advocate, North Carolina

Sarah Wise Miller
Cancer Advocate, New York

David Perry, Esq.
Attorney, K & L Gates LLP, California

William J. Perry
CEO, The Perry Strategy Group, California

*Denise L. Richards
Actress, California

Lois Stulberg
Community Leader, Michigan

*Nicholas J. Vogelzang, MD
Comprehensive Cancer Centers, Nevada

Christopher G. Wood, MD, FACS
Department of Urology, M. D. Anderson Cancer Center, Texas

*non-voting director

The Medical Advisory Board Steering Committee of the Kidney Cancer Association

Michael B. Atkins, MD
Georgetown University School of Medicine

Ronald M. Bukowski, MD, *Co-Chair*
Bukowski Consulting, LLC
Cleveland Clinic Taussig Cancer Institute

Toni Choueiri, MD, *Co-Chair*
Dana-Farber Cancer Institute

Bernard Escudier, MD
Institut Gustave-Roussy, Villejuif

James Hsieh, MD
Memorial Sloan-Kettering Cancer Center

Thomas Hutson, DO, PharmD, FACP
Baylor University Medical Center

Bradley Leibovich, MD
Mayo Clinic Cancer Cente

Walter Stadler, MD
University of Chicago Medical Center

Nizar Tannir, MD
M.D. Anderson Cancer Center

Christopher G. Wood, MD
M.D. Anderson Cancer Center

Kidney Cancer Association Staff

Carolyn E. Konosky
President

William P. Bro
Secretary

Notes On The Text

Both science and technology change rapidly, and developments in the treatment of kidney cancer in the years following publication of this booklet are likely. This may make the text less up-to-date. More recent information may be available over the Internet. Changes in the addresses, telephone numbers, and Internet sites of the organizations listed in this booklet are to be expected, and we apologize for any inconvenience they may cause.

EDITORIAL: Paul Larson Communications
DESIGN: McGuire Associates
02-2017 1-M

TABLE OF CONTENTS

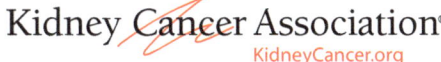

Kidney Cancer Association®
KidneyCancer.org

Kidney Cancer Association
Phone: 1-800-850-9132
www.kidneycancer.org
office@kidneycancer.org

Lessons for Living Well

"I'm living, and not only that, I'm living well." My statement may not seem particularly remarkable. But in 2000, when I was diagnosed with Stage III kidney cancer and given less than a year to live, making such a statement would have seemed unimaginable to me. In the sixteen years since receiving that shattering death sentence, I have often felt like an unwilling passenger on a harrowing roller coaster ride. However, along the way I have learned some valuable lessons—lessons that I believe have not only kept me alive, but have kept me living well.

Within six months of my diagnosis, my cancer had metastasized to my lungs and brain. If I had taken as gospel the words and statistics of the generalist who pronounced my sentence, I would not be here today. After recovering from the initial shock, I made a decisive commitment to live. I educated myself about my disease. I read everything about kidney cancer that I could get my hands on, most of which I found on the Internet. My research led me to seek out a specialist in kidney cancer, who led me to another specialist, who led me to another. Not only did these amazing doctors possess expert knowledge about my disease, but equally important, their optimism and encouragement helped me to manage my fear and hold fast to the commitment to live that I had made to myself.

Over the years, I have experienced the gamut of conditions, complications, and side effects. I have participated in clinical trials, and I have moved from therapy to therapy—eight of them at last count. Thanks to the exciting advances being made in kidney cancer research, I have learned that there is always another possible treatment option—another "plan B, C, and D" in the pipeline, as my oncologist likes to tell me. Indeed, as I have learned in so many ways, there is always a reason to stay positive.

The more I have learned, the more optimistic I have become. My life partner, Cindy, has steadfastly shared in my optimism, as have my family members and friends. I have become convinced that having a caring expert in kidney cancer sharing in my fight is absolutely vital to my physical, mental, and emotional well-being.

And so, sixteen years later, I'm living, and not only that, I'm living well. Equipped with expert medical care, a loving support system, an expanding horizon of new research and therapy, a thriving online kidney cancer community, a fair bit of courage, and a huge dose of optimism, I expect to be living well for many years to come.

CHAPTER 1

INTRODUCTION

"I have kidney cancer. What now?"

Your doctor has just told you that you have cancer. Your mind whirls with emotion. Suddenly, you are facing a health crisis. Now, more than ever, you need to think clearly, despite strong emotions.

This book contains information from scientists, physicians and other health professionals who are experts in understanding and treating kidney cancer. The goal of this book is to help you face the challenge of kidney cancer by helping you become better informed.

Your ability to think, to use information, and to make choices about treatment can help bend the odds in your favor. Reading this book is the first step.

This section provides you with brief background information about kidney cancer and some immediate resources that may

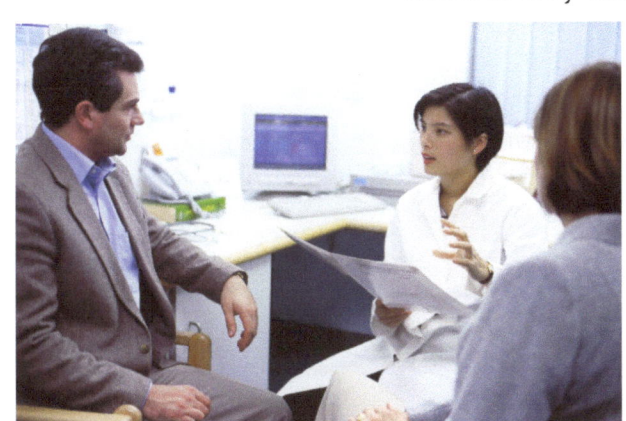

An initial diagnosis of kidney cancer can be difficult. But with support and good information, you can face the challenge.

be helpful. The chapters that follow provide more in-depth information, ranging from current surgical and therapeutic approaches to practical advice for living with cancer day to day.

Improving your health starts right now!

You Are Not Alone

Kidney cancer is among the 10 most common cancers in both men and women. Overall, the lifetime risk for developing kidney cancer is about 1 in 63 (1.6%). The National Cancer Institute estimates that more than 60,000 people are diagnosed with kidney cancer annually. Still, there is hope: An estimated 375,925 kidney cancer survivors are living in the United States right now. Recent advances in diagnosis, surgical procedures, and treatment options will allow even more patients to live with the disease, continuing to maintain their normal schedules and lifestyles.

2005 marked the beginning of an important new era for kidney cancer patients, with the approval by the Food and Drug Administration (FDA) of the first oral drug to treat this disease. A second drug was approved in early 2006. A third drug was approved in 2007, three additional drugs were approved in 2009, and two more new drugs were approved in 2012 and 2016. These drugs, which are discussed later in this book, target cancer cells in different ways than previous drugs used to treat kidney cancer, and will have a very positive impact for many patients. Hence, the name "targeted therapies" was given to this class of medications. Continued research efforts will improve our understanding of the disease even more and increase the options available to fight kidney cancer.

Each person diagnosed with kidney cancer goes through the shock of being told they have the disease. It is a difficult experience. Feelings of disbelief, loneliness, alienation, fear, frustration, anger, and hurt are natural parts of any life- threatening illness. It is okay to have these feelings, to cry, and to be upset.

After your diagnosis, it's time to start healing. Don't let your emotions and your cancer damage your home life or relations with the important people in your life. They may also be hurting inside, fearing for you and themselves. When cancer strikes, it hits the whole family. Your friends and family will play an important role as you fight this disease.

Let's Begin

Sometimes kidney cancer is called by its medical name, renal cell carcinoma. Renal is from the Latin word renalis for kidneys. Kidney cancer appears in various forms, including clear cell, papillary, sarcomatoid, transitional cell, and others. These will be explained in more detail later in this book.

Some patients are diagnosed before the cancer has metastasized (spread) to other parts of the body, while others have metastatic disease when their cancer is initially diagnosed. If patients have metastatic disease, either surgery or systemic medical therapy – that is, a treatment that is injected into the bloodstream or swallowed – may be recommended first, depending on the patient's situation. If surgery is done first, additional treatment may be recommended to treat metastatic disease or to delay the cancer's return.

The choice of treatment, where treatment is administered, the frequency of check-ups, and many other aspects of the management of your disease are determined with input from you. The more you know, the better your decisions, and the more you can feel in control of your illness. Knowledge about your disease will help you better communicate with your doctor and nurse, and increase your confidence in the treatment that you receive. Getting smarter about kidney cancer is an important step in effectively fighting your disease.

How to Learn More About Kidney Cancer

Your Doctor

Your own doctor can be one of the best sources of information about your disease and its treatment. Doctors who specialize in treating cancer are known as oncologists. After an initial diagnosis is made, don't be afraid to ask your doctor many questions. You should also consider getting a second opinion from another doctor who is a kidney cancer specialist. If you do not know the name of a specialist, you may obtain names from the Kidney Cancer Association (email the request via the Association's website at www.kidneycancer.org or by calling 1-800-850-9132). Your doctor should not be offended if you seek a second opinion. It is common practice. In fact, your doctor often gives second opinions to other patients and to colleagues. You may not need to have tests repeated because often the results of your previous tests can be sent to the second doctor. Rarely will a second opinion change your diagnosis, but it can give you useful information and fresh insights about treatment alternatives. In addition, your insurance company may require a second opinion. If you are in a health mainte-nance organization (HMO), you should find out about its policy concerning second opinions. You'll find more information about working with your doctor in the chapter of this booklet titled "Patient Empowerment."

The Kidney Cancer Association

The Kidney Cancer Association is available to assist you in many ways, including providing written information on the disease, treatment options, and resources. You can contact the Kidney Cancer Association at 1-800-850-9132, or visit its web-site at www.kidneycancer.org. The Kidney Cancer Association's website has valuable information that you can read, print, or share with family and friends.

A special note about this book

"We Have Kidney Cancer" is an essential resource for kidney

cancer patients. Now in its fifth printing, the book is updated every few years. While this book offers the most current information about kidney cancer at the time of its printing, it is possible that new information and treatments may now be available and are not part of this edition. For that reason it is always a good idea to check the Kidney Cancer Association website for the latest information and updates that might be important. An electronic version of "We Have Kidney Cancer" is available at the website and any updated sections of the book are clearly marked.

Other Patients

Kidney cancer patients can learn a great deal from one another. The best way to do that is to attend a patient meeting sponsored by the Kidney Cancer Association or support groups sponsored by your local hospital. Support groups provide excellent open environments for frank exchange with other patients and professional counselors.

The National Cancer Information Service

No matter where you live in the United States, you can call 1-800-4-CANCER, the toll-free telephone number of the National Cancer Information Service. You can also contact the information service through its website at www.cancer.gov/contact/contact-center. This information service is provided by the National Cancer Institute, which is part of the National Institutes of Health (NIH). The NIH is operated by the U.S. Department of Health and Human Services. You can ask for a variety of free booklets.

Other Websites

There are many other websites that can help you understand the disease and its diagnosis, treatment options, dealing with the illness and side effects of treatment, work, and coping with a life-threatening diagnosis. A list of trusted websites is included later in this book (Chapter 11). You must be careful because some medical information on the Internet is posted by nonprofessionals and is not reliable. Always check the site to learn more about the source of any information provided. Look for well-known, established sources online and don't rely on just one website. Reputable sites with reliable information for patients are sometimes accredited (approved) by a governing body such as "Health on the NET." In any case, use common sense and compare sites carefully when considering online material.

Libraries

More and more research is being done as scientists and physicians gain new knowledge about how kidney cancer develops and spreads, in order to improve our ability to treat and cure more patients. Nursing literature may be helpful to understand the treatment options and management of side effects. A reference library may be able to help with a medical literature search if this interests you.

A simple paperback medical dictionary can help you understand many of the terms and abbreviations you will encounter as you learn more about kidney cancer. Check your local bookstore

New Research from Conferences and Meetings

The amount of research on kidney cancer being presented at national and international physician and nursing conferences and published literature reporting research results has increased significantly in recent years. There are many meetings devoted to education and open dialogue, and researchers are continually discovering new information about kidney cancer. Doctors and nurses will provide you with information about recent research findings as they discuss treatment options and care during the course of your treatment.

What Caused your Kidney Cancer?

Most cancers are related to chance events. Mutations in individual cells result in disordered cell growth. But some external factors, such as smoking and obesity, have also been related to a higher incidence of kidney cancer. In an attempt to answer the question "Why me?" some people want to identify such factors as a cause for their cancer. Although it is important for people to know what factors or behaviors are associated with an increased risk of kidney cancer, blaming yourself for past behavior is neither helpful nor healing. The fact that a person's behavior included a risk factor such as smoking doesn't necessarily mean the factor caused the cancer.

Inherited Kidney Cancer

Genetic factors have been linked to an increased risk of developing kidney cancer. For example, a hereditary disorder called von Hippel-Lindau (VHL) disease is associated with a high risk of developing kidney cancer. Scientists have isolated the gene responsible for VHL disease, and this discovery offers exciting future possibilities for improved diagnosis and treatment of some kidney cancers. Another genetic mutation thought to be associated with RCC is tuberous sclerosis. It is a disease characterized by small tumors of the blood vessels that results in numerous bumps on the skin, mental retardation, seizures, and cysts in the kidneys, liver, and pancreas. The Birt-Hogg-Dubé syndrome is another disorder associated with kidney cancer that is characterized by the presence of multiple small bumps (nodules) on the skin covering the nose, cheeks, forehead, ears, and neck.

Information and Understanding

As you learn more about kidney cancer, keep an open mind. Our knowledge and understanding about the disease are constantly changing, and some of the information you may read on the Internet or from other sources may be outdated or inaccurate. If you have questions about anything you read, be sure to ask your health care team. They can give you up-to-date information. Asking questions is a very important way to reduce fear and anxiety and is the only way to truly empower yourself to make the best decisions regarding treatment for your kidney cancer.

Doctors and nurses will be very willing to answer your questions, because the more you understand, the better you will be able to participate as an active member of your health-care team.

We think that learning more about the disease and your treatment choices will help you.

What Kidneys Do

The kidneys are located on each side of your body, toward the back, at the bottom of your rib cage. They are surrounded by fatty tissue, which serves to cushion and protect them. An adrenal gland is located on the top of each kidney. Kidneys come in pairs but you can live a normal life with only one kidney.

Each kidney weighs about 8 ounces and measures 4 to 5 inches long by 2 to 3 inches wide. The adult kidney is curved in the shape of a kidney bean with an indentation in the center where the renal artery, renal vein, and ureter connect. Blood enters the kidney through the renal artery and exits through the renal vein. The main job of the kidneys is to filter the blood and cleanse the body of waste products such as urea, excess salt, and other substances. The fluid which the kidneys excrete and which contains these dissolved waste products is called urine. The urine drains through the ureter, a long, slender tube connecting the kidney to the bladder.

The kidney is encased in a membrane called the capsule. This membrane is flexible and stretches when a tumor is formed inside the kidney. If diagnosed early, the tumor may remain inside the capsule and can be more easily treated by surgical removal of the kidney. Early diagnosis is aided by knowing the symptoms of kidney cancer and seeing your doctor as soon as possible.

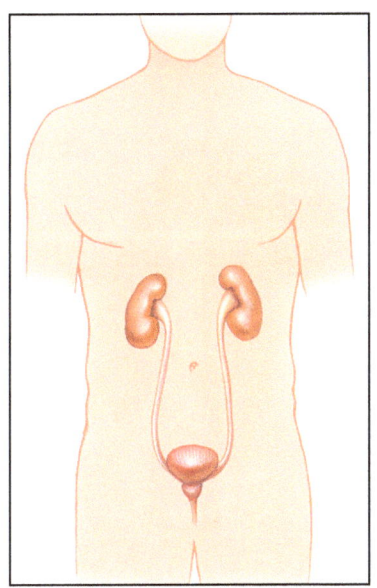

Location of the kidneys
in the body

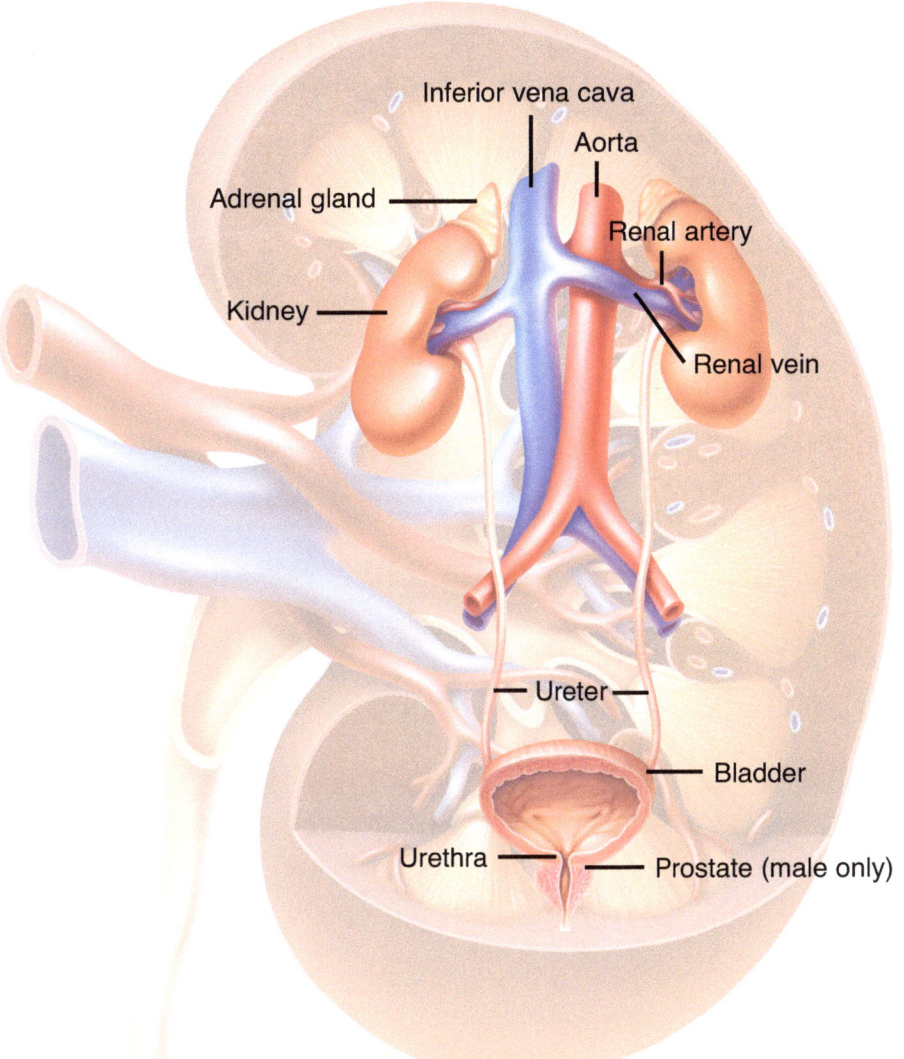

Find the best medical team you can

"Finding the right medical team makes a big difference. When my husband was diagnosed, we were shocked. Our doctor said there was probably very little that could be done because it was so advanced and he estimated my husband had nine months to live. But he put us in touch with another doctor who knew more about kidney cancer and that was the beginning of finding our current medical team.

The second doctor referred us to a very large, well known medical clinic that specialized in kidney cancer. After surgery to remove his kidney, my husband started a clinical trial with high-dose Interleukin 2 and Peg-Intron shots three times a week. For 18 months he was stable, but the tumors started to grow, so he went on a second trial. When those treatments stopped being effective he went into another trial. The medical team has helped him move into the new trials and they have been wonderful.

As a retired nurse, I know the things that can lead to worry in medical care. But if you have the right team and the right hospital it helps take away the worry. Our team explains everything to us and always has an option if a course of treatment doesn't work out. They monitor my husband very closely and they answer all of our questions – and that makes you feel a lot better."

CHAPTER 2

UNDERSTANDING KIDNEY CANCER

A comprehensive look at types, symptoms, treatments, and much more…Use this section to formulate questions for your doctor about the status of your kidney cancer.

According to the American Cancer Society (ACS), over 1.6 million new cases of cancer are diagnosed each year in the United States. In recent years, the percentage of cases involving kidney cancer have made up less than 4% of the total. The ACS estimated in 2015 that more than 60,000 of the new cancer cases are individuals diagnosed with kidney cancer.

Kidney cancer occurs roughly twice as often in men as in women, but the gap is narrowing. The American Cancer Society estimated in 2016 that just over 14,000 people die annually from the disease. However, it is also estimated that more than 375,000 kidney cancer survivors are living in the United States right now. These statistics include both adults and children and include all forms of kidney cancer.

Renal cell carcinoma (RCC) is the most common type of kidney cancer. In terms of all cancers, renal cell carcinoma is relatively rare. It is usually treated initially with surgery to remove the tumor. If caught in early stages, the chance that it will return is low. Unfortunately, it has few symptoms in its early stages, so it is usually undiagnosed or misdiagnosed and not detected until the tumor has grown fairly large. At that point, it displaces other nearby organs, causing symptoms. Increasingly, many kidney (renal) tumors are found incidentally on x-rays or ultrasound examinations performed for reasons that don't relate to the tumor or any of its potential symptoms.

There are several risk factors associated with the development of kidney cancer. These include: smoking, which almost doubles one's risk; obesity; and exposure to toxic chemicals such as asbestos, cadmium and petroleum by-products (gasoline, for example). Having family members with kidney cancer also increases one's risk.

The most common symptom of kidney cancer is painless urination of blood, a condition known as hematuria. This symptom occurs in 20% to 25% of patients. Often, blood in the urine will occur one day and not the next. (Note that blood in the urine can indicate other diseases besides kidney cancer, such as kidney stones or infection. When blood in the urine does occur, a doctor should evaluate this symptom immediately.)

Other common symptoms of kidney cancer include the presence of an abdominal mass, a hard lump or a thickening or bulging under the skin that can be seen or felt as the tumor grows. There also may be back or flank pain or pressure. Kidney cancer occurs most often in individuals between the age of 40 and 60. Since back pain is common among people over 40 years of age, such pain is often ignored and the presence of kidney cancer can go undetected.

If the tumor has spread to distant organs, symptoms may vary, depending on the specific organ affected, though patients may notice unexplained weight loss, fevers, anemia, or high blood pressure.

Even if your cancer originates in the kidney and spreads to other organs, it is still considered kidney cancer. The following list includes symptoms and/or signs in patients at the time of their diagnosis. Note that some patients don't show symptoms:

> **Blood in the urine**
> **Abdominal mass**
> **Back or flank pain**
> **Weight loss**
> **Low blood counts (anemia)**
> **Tumor calcification on x-ray**
> **Symptoms of metastases**
> **Fever**
> **High calcium in blood**

Subtypes of Renal Cell Carcinoma (RCC)

Not all kidney cancers are the same. There is an increasing understanding among clinicians and researchers that there are different subtypes of RCC and that they behave quite differently, both with regard to how aggressive they are in the patient and how they respond to treatment. Ten or fifteen years ago, it was common for a pathology report from a patient with kidney cancer to read simply "Renal Cell Carcinoma." This simple diagnosis is now thought to be incomplete. Identification of the specific subtype or cell type (histology) of the kidney cancer can be as important in determining the chance for recovery (known as prognosis) as knowing the stage or grade of the RCC. Your doctor should give you information regarding the histology, grade, and stage of your kidney cancer. If not, you should feel comfortable asking for this information since it is an important part of your treatment planning.

The subtypes of RCC come from the description of the cell's appearance and other characteristics. They include:

Clear Cell (conventional) RCC

This is the most common form of kidney cancer and represents between 66% and 75% of all cases. Clear cell RCC is the cell type associated with the von Hippel-Lindau (VHL) gene mutation in hereditary kidney cancer. In fact, approximately 70% of non-hereditary cases of clear cell RCC also have a VHL mutation. Much of today's research, which is attempting to identify new effective treatments for patients with locally advanced or metastatic disease, is focused on this disease sub-type since it is the most common type of RCC. When the tumor has not spread, prognosis can be very good following surgical excision (removal of the tumor). Prognosis for the patient is directly related to both the cancer's stage (tumor size and rate of growth) and grade (the characteristics of a tumor's cell structure). Staging and grading are both explained later in this chapter. Patients with metastatic clear cell RCC – or a tumor that has spread to other parts of the body – have a poorer prognosis.

Papillary RCC

This is the second most common form of kidney cancer, making up approximately 15% of cases. Papillary RCC itself is divided into two subtypes based on cell appearance: Type I (5%) and Type II (10%). There is an increased incidence of papillary RCC in African Americans and an increased incidence of bilateral disease (involving both kidneys) associated with this subtype. There are also hereditary forms of both Type I and Type II papillary RCC. When papillary RCC has not spread, surgical removal is usually associated with an excellent prognosis. Targeted therapies are modestly effective based on several randomized clinical trials, with Sutent® (sunitinib) and Afinitor® (everolimus) being the primary choices for treatment. Participation in a clinical trial should be strongly considered.

Chromophobe RCC

This rare form of kidney cancer represents approximately 5% of RCC cases. This type of RCC is thought to originate from the same cell type as those that form renal oncocytomas (see below). Hybrid tumors that contain features of both chromophobe RCC and renal oncocytoma have also been diagnosed. There is a familial or inherited form of chromophobe RCC (in association with renal oncocytoma) called Birt-Hogg-Dubé syndrome, which is also associated with a specific genetic mutation. Chromophobe RCC rarely metastasizes until very late in its clinical course, and surgical removal of localized or even locally advanced disease is usually associated with an excellent prognosis. Metastatic chromophobe RCC is quite rare, and no standard therapy currently exists.

Renal Oncocytoma

This is a benign tumor of the kidney that makes up approximately 5% of all kidney tumors. These tumors do not metastasize, although they can grow to a large size in the kidney and invade local structures, which can result in symptoms requiring surgery. They are thought to be related to chromophobe RCC, and it can be quite difficult to differentiate the two. The tumor is treated by a partial or complete removal of the kidney.

Unclassified RCC

Less than 1% of renal cell carcinomas are an unclassified type. They don't fit into one of the more common subtypes of RCC listed above. When examined under a microscope, these unclassified cancer cells have a structure and genetic features that don't match the description of the more common RCC subtypes. This category usually includes aggressive tumors that do not respond to traditional therapy for RCC.

Translocation Carcinomas

A distinct variant of RCC, referred to as translocation carcinoma, is associated with fusion of the TFE3 gene to a number of other genes on chromosome Xp11.2. Translocation carcinoma tends to occur at a younger age compared with other forms of kidney cancer. In one series of 54 patients, the median age was 24 years, and the disease was more common in women than in men (57% vs. 43%). Translocation carcinoma has also been reported in children who have received antecedent chemotherapy for malignancies, autoimmune disorders, or bone marrow transplant conditioning.

Collecting Duct Carcinoma

This is a rare and very aggressive variant of kidney cancer that represents less than 1% of cases. This form of RCC is usually metastatic at the time of diagnosis, and is more common in younger individuals. Treatment has been directed at using chemotherapy-based regimens, similar to those used in the treatment of transitional cell carcinoma (see below), as these tumors do not respond to traditional RCC therapies such as immunotherapy.

Medullary RCC

This is also a very rare and aggressive variant of kidney cancer, thought to be a variant of collecting duct carcinoma. It is commonly associated with the sickle cell trait, and therefore is more common in the African-American population. It represents less than 1% of all kidney cancers diagnosed. Chemotherapy remains the main focus of treatment for this disease.

Sarcomatoid RCC

This condition is characterized by a poorly differentiated tumor, and can occur with any of the common RCC subtypes. The term refers to the fact that the RCC cells – when viewed under the microscope – have the appearance of sarcoma cells. The percentage of sarcomatoid differentiation is usually reflected in the tumor's pathology report and relates to the tumor's aggressiveness. The prognosis associated with sarcomatoid RCC was once thought to be uniformly poor, but now there is more hope of treatment with the availability of new drugs. The condition is found frequently in patients whose kidney cancer has metastasized widely. This form of kidney cancer is sometimes treated with chemotherapy.

Transitional Cell Carcinoma of the Kidney

Transitional cell carcinoma (TCC) of the kidney is a rare and potentially very aggressive tumor that should not be considered a true kidney cancer, but instead should be grouped with bladder cancer. If the cancer has not spread, the tumor can be treated by surgical removal of both the kidney and its ureter, although recurrences of TCC in the bladder are common. When the tumor is large or has metastasized, the prognosis is poor, and treatment options are similar to those for metastatic urinary bladder cancer, which include chemotherapy.

Detection, Diagnosis and Staging

Because kidney cancer may spread to other parts of the body, it is important to be very thorough in testing for its presence. All approaches begin with a careful physical examination, combined with a complete discussion of past and present medical problems. Your doctor may order some or all of the following tests to determine the extent of your cancer and to develop your treatment plan.

Computed Tomography (CT scan)

A CT scan, commonly called a "CAT" scan, is a highly specialized test that is used to visualize internal organs and provides a very accurate picture of specific areas of the body. It is used as one of the primary imaging tools for the assessment of RCC. If the initial sign of the tumor is a mass or thickening in the kidney area detected on an x-ray taken for other reasons, or seen or felt during a physical exam, a CT scan is often ordered.

CT scans are more detailed than ordinary x-rays, taking pictures of your organs one thin slice at a time from different angles. Then a computer puts the images together to show the size and location of any abnormalities. To enhance the image of the abdominal organs, a barium solution may be taken orally (by mouth) before the scan. An IV may also be placed for injection of additional contrast dye. There is generally no pain associated with the CT scan, although the IV dye (also called IV contrast) may cause a hot, flushing sensation. Some people may also experience an allergic reaction to IV dye, especially individuals who are allergic to iodine. Depending on the part of the body visualized, dietary restrictions may be required prior to the procedure. Sometimes the IV contrast will not be given if the kidney function is not within a certain range based on the creatinine level. Some radiology departments use the estimated glomerular filtration rate (eGFR) to determine if there is sufficient kidney function for IV contrast administration.

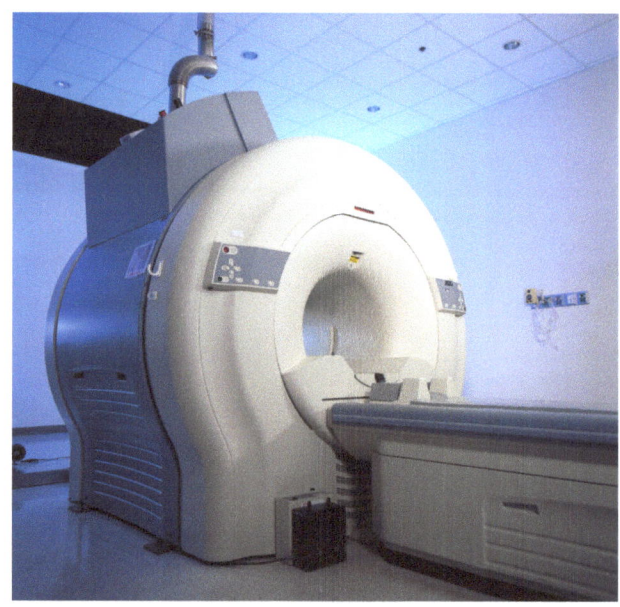

A typical CT scanner. Magnetic Resonance Imaging (MRI) and Computed Tomography (CT) are common tests used in the diagnosis of kidney cancer.

Magnetic Resonance Imaging (MRI)

An MRI is a highly specialized scan that is similar to a CT scan, but may be better suited for assessing certain areas of the body, such as the bones, brain or spine. It creates an accurate cross-section picture of specific organs within the body, to allow for a layer-by-layer examination. An MRI is usually not a painful procedure. Because it uses a powerful magnet to produce the images, people with metal within their body – such as prosthetic hip replacements, pacemakers, or metal plates – should discuss the use of an MRI with their doctor and the MRI technician before the scan is performed. The test may require the patient to lie still for a long time, usually in a narrow space, which may be difficult for some people who do not like closed-in spaces. MRI scans are often used in cases where CT scans may not be able to view an area of the body well enough. The type of IV contrast used for MRI scans is gadolinium, with the same precautions regarding renal function.

Bone Scan

A bone scan can be used to check for the spread of cancer to the bones. It is done by injecting small amounts of a special radioactive material through a vein into your bloodstream. This material is carried to the bone, where it collects in areas where there is a lot of bone activity. The test can identify both cancerous and non-cancerous diseases, but the test can't distinguish between cancer and other conditions such as arthritis when used alone. In some cases, RCC in bone does not show up on a bone scan. Therefore other tests may be needed, such as x-rays or CT scans.

Positron Emission Tomography (PET) Scan

A PET scan is a very specialized diagnostic study that provides information about how extensively a cancer has spread, based on certain activities of the cells. PET scans are typically used for breast, colorectal, ovarian, lymphoma, lung, melanoma, and head and neck cancer. The effectiveness of PET scans for kidney cancer is still being studied.

Unlike CT and MRI scans, which produce images of internal organs or other structures, a PET scan produces images based on the chemical and physiological changes related to a cell's metabolism. This is important because chemical and physiological changes in the cells often occur before structural changes in tissues can be seen. As a result, PET scans can help distinguish benign from malignant tumors and help doctors determine the stage of cancer spread in the patient. PET scans can also measure whether or not treatment therapies are working. PET scans are quite often used in combination with CT and MRI scans. A PET scan can last from 15 minutes to two hours, depending on the area of the body being scanned.

Ultrasonography (Ultrasound or US)

If there is blood in the urine, an ultrasound of the abdomen with special attention to the kidneys, ureters, and bladder may be ordered. US can also be used to help distinguish between a cyst and a solid mass. Usually no preparation is needed for this test, and it is generally not uncomfortable. It utilizes sound waves to produce images of internal organs, helping the radiologist detect any masses that may be present. A wand called a transducer is passed over the skin, and emits sound waves that are detected as echoes bouncing back off internal organs. The echo-pattern images produced by kidney tumors look different from those of normal kidney tissue. This test may be used for initial diagnosis of a kidney mass or to help visualize a mass when a fine needle biopsy is done (see Biopsy Procedure below).

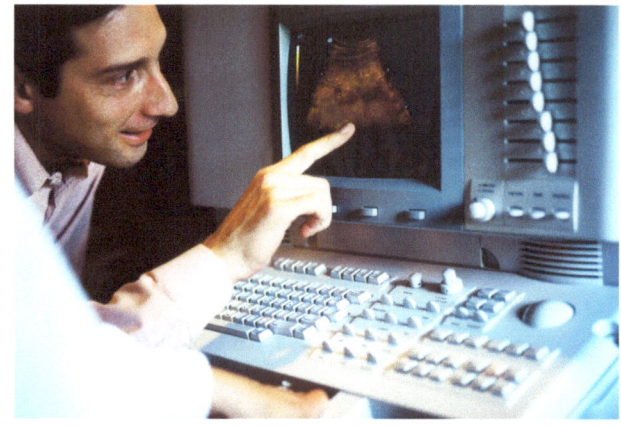
Ultrasound testing may be used to help diagnose kidney cancer.

Intravenous Pyelogram (IVP)

An IVP test may be used. Special dye is injected into a blood vessel, usually in the arm. The dye circulates through the bloodstream to the different organs of the body, including the kidneys. X-rays are taken of the kidneys as the dye circulates through them. This will identify any abnormalities within the kidney. If either the ultrasound or IVP is abnormal, a CT scan may be ordered.

Chest X-ray

An x-ray of the chest may be done to see if the cancer has spread to the lungs. If something is seen on the x-ray, the doctor may order a CT scan of the chest to help determine what it is.

Biopsy Procedure

If, after diagnostic tests are completed, there is a strong clinical suspicion that the kidney mass is cancerous (malignant), surgical removal of all or part of the kidney (nephrectomy) will be performed immediately. In certain situations a biopsy of the mass may be performed, but this is not common. During a biopsy procedure, a small sample of tissue is removed from the mass and examined to determine whether it is benign or malignant. There are several ways to perform a biopsy of a kidney mass, though the most common method is a procedure called a fine needle aspiration (FNA) or fine needle biopsy. Using ultrasound or a CT scanner for guidance, the doctor will insert a long, thin needle through the skin, directly into the mass, and remove the sample tissue. A pathologist will evaluate the biopsy tissue under a microscope to determine whether it is benign or malignant. If it is malignant, the pathologist also will identify the histology, or cell type.

If there is clear evidence of widespread metastasis at the time of the discovery of the kidney mass, a biopsy may be taken from an area of metastasis, instead of from the kidney. This may be recommended to reduce risk of bleeding if the metastatic area is more easily accessible than the kidney. A biopsy can help in planning subsequent therapy and treatment options, even though the diagnosis is not in question.

Other Tests

In addition to the tests described above, your doctor may order one or more of the following lab tests to complete your evaluation.

Urinalysis

Urinalysis is usually part of a complete physical exam. Microscopic and chemical tests are performed that will detect small amounts of blood and other substances not seen with the naked eye.

About half of all patients with renal cell cancer will have blood in their urine.

Blood tests

A complete blood count and chemical test of the blood can detect findings associated with RCC. Anemia (too few red blood cells) is very common. Erythrocytosis (too many red blood cells) may also occur because some of these renal cancers produce a hormone (erythropoietin) that can increase red blood cell production by the bone marrow.

High levels of liver-function enzymes in the blood (for reasons not known) and hypercalcemia (high calcium levels) sometimes occur.

The Role of Staging and Grading

Staging of a cancer is the process of classifying how far a cancer has spread, while **grading** determines the characteristics and makeup of the cancer's cells. The two systems play different roles, but both staging and grading are important predictors of the course of the disease and treatment effectiveness (prognosis). They are useful in determining what therapy is appropriate and the chance of treatment success.

Staging

Certain imaging tests, including CT and MRI scans, can help to detect whether the cancer has spread to certain organs and to determine staging. Blood tests will also be done to evaluate your overall health.

A staging system is a standardized way in which the cancer care team describes the extent of the cancer. The most commonly used staging system was developed by the American Joint Committee on Cancer (AJCC).

American Joint Committee on Cancer (AJCC) TNM Staging System

The AJCC staging system is based on the evaluation of the tumor size on the kidney (T), lymph node involvement (whether or not the cancer has spread to the nearby lymph nodes) (N), and the extent of metastasis (whether or not the cancer has spread to distant areas of the body) (M). Evaluation of the T, N, and M components is followed by a stage grouping.

The T component relates to the size of the primary tumor. The numerical value increases with tumor size and extent of invasiveness. The letter T followed by a number from 0 to 4 describes the tumor's size and spread to nearby tissues. Some of these numbers are further subdivided with letters, such as T1a and T1b. Higher T numbers indicate a larger tumor and/or more extensive spread to tissues near the kidney.

The N component designates the presence or absence of tumor in nearby lymph nodes. Lymph nodes are bean-sized structures with collections of immune cells (lymphocytes) that help fight infections and cancers. The letter N followed by a number from 0 to 2 indicates whether the cancer has spread to lymph nodes near the kidney and, if so, how many are affected.

The M component identifies how far the cancer has spread from the primary tumor. The letter **M** followed by a 0 or 1 indicates whether or not the cancer has spread to distant organs such as the lungs or bones, or to lymph nodes that are in other parts of the body.

Detailed Definitions of T, N, and M Categories

Primary tumor (T):

TX: Primary tumor cannot be evaluated.

T0: No evidence of a primary tumor.

T1s: Carcinoma in situ (early cancer that has not spread to neighboring tissue).

T1-T4: Each level (1-4) indicates the size and/or extent of the primary tumor.

Regional lymph nodes (N):

NX: Regional lymph nodes cannot be evaluated.

N0: No regional lymph node involvement (no cancer found in the lymph nodes).

N1-N3: Each level (1-3) indicates involvement of regional lymph nodes (number and/or extent of spread).

Extent of Metastasis (M):

M0: No distant metastasis (cancer has not spread to other parts of the body).

M1: Distant metastasis (cancer has spread to distant parts of the body).

Renal Cell Cancer Stage Grouping

Stage I: The tumor is 7 cm or smaller and limited to the kidney. There is no spread to lymph nodes or distant organs.

Stage II: The tumor is larger than 7 cm but is still limited to the kidney. There is no spread to lymph nodes or distant organs.

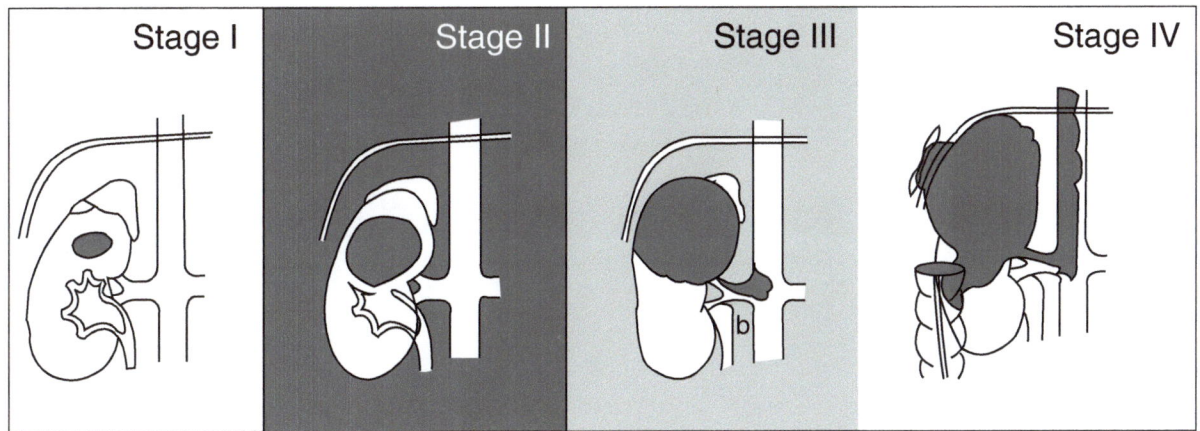

Stage III: This stage includes any tumor that has spread to only one nearby lymph node but not to other organs. Stage III also includes tumors that have not spread to lymph nodes or distant organs but have spread to the adrenal glands, to fatty tissue around the kidney, and/or have grown into the large vein (vena cava) leading from the kidney to the heart.

Stage IV: This stage includes any cancers that have spread directly through the fatty tissue and beyond Gerota's fascia, the fibrous tissue that surrounds the kidney. Stage IV also includes any cancer that has spread to more than one lymph node near the kidney, or to any lymph node distant from the kidney, or to any distant organs such as the lungs, bone, or brain.

Grading

The system for determining the characteristics of cancer cells is called Fuhrman grading. The Fuhrman grade is determined by a pathologist, who will review the cellular details of the tumor. The grade is based on an examination of how closely the cancer cell's nucleus (part of a cell in which DNA is stored) resembles a normal kidney cell's nucleus.

Kidney cancers are usually given a Fuhrman grade on a scale of 1 through 4. Grade 1 kidney cancers have cell nuclei that look very much like a normal kidney cell nucleus. These cancers are usually slow-growing and are slow to spread to other parts of the body. They tend to have a good outlook (prognosis). Grade 4 kidney cancer, on the upper end of the Fuhrman scale, looks quite different from normal kidney cells and has a less favorable prognosis. Generally, the higher the Fuhrman grade, the less favorable the prognosis.

It is important to note that while predictions can be made based on grading and staging, prognosis can vary widely, even within Stage I and often in Stage IV. You should always consult with your doctor, who will help provide an accurate assessment of the course of your disease.

NOTES

With Surgery and Improved Follow-up Treatment, There's Hope

Patient: Beverly
Age: 67

"I had my nephrectomy 14 years ago. At the time my husband and I were living in the Philippines. I came back to the United States and had the surgery here, at Johns Hopkins.

The surgery itself was very straightforward. I had a radical nephrectomy and a good outcome, fortunately, as the tumor had not metastasized.

I was a little frustrated in recovery because unlike other patients on my floor, I was unable to get up and start walking around right away. It was too painful for the first couple of days. My rib cage was very sensitive. But fairly soon I was able to get up and start moving and my daughters then really pushed me to get some exercise every day. I think this helped move my recovery along. Sitting at the table for a meal was a little difficult for awhile, but gradually that pain went away too. Within six weeks I was able to travel back to the Philippines.

I now volunteer as a kidney cancer patient advocate and in the Cancer Patient Education Program at the medical center in my home city. My advice for kidney cancer patients has always been to remain hopeful, but with new drug developments over the last few years, there is more reason to be hopeful than ever before. To know that there is finally an effective treatment through the new approved medications brings tremendous room for optimism. Kidney cancer doesn't have to be the dire prognosis that it used to be."

CHAPTER 3

SURGICAL TREATMENT

Understanding the various surgical approaches to the most common form of kidney cancer

Surgery is considered the primary treatment for most kidney cancers. A variety of surgical procedures are available, depending on the type, size of tumor, extent of disease, and the patient's overall physical condition. Your doctor will discuss the surgical options that are appropriate for you.

Traditional Surgery: Removing All or Part of the Kidney

Traditionally, the most common treatment of most kidney cancers begins with removal of the primary tumor in an operation called a nephrectomy. In some cases this requires complete removal of the kidney (radical nephrectomy); in other cases, only part of the kidney is removed (partial nephrectomy). The purpose of surgery is to remove the primary tumor and involved

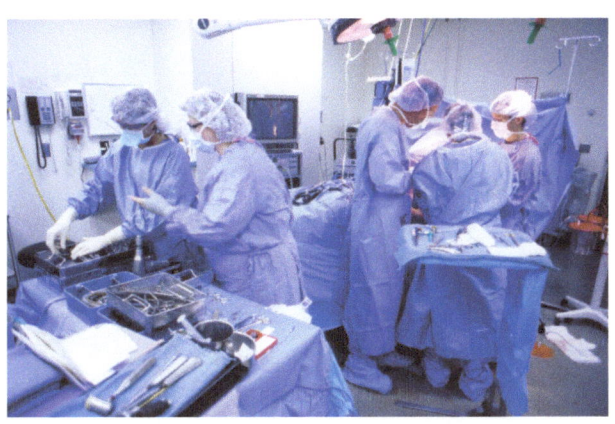

Full or partial nephrectomy is considered the primary treatment for most kidney cancers.

tissue in the kidney. Thousands of nephrectomies are performed every year for kidney cancer as well as for other diseases. Although it is a major surgery, the potential risks are well defined and it is usually quite safe if you do not have any underlying illnesses, such as heart disease or liver disease. Complications are not common unless the tumor is locally advanced, such as when the tumor extends into the renal vein or inferior vena cava (the large vein through which blood from your legs and internal organs returns to the heart), or the tumor has spread beyond the kidney.

Extension of the tumor into the vein requires blood vessel surgery to remove the tumor from the vein or even the vein itself. This condition is familiar to most surgeons, but it prolongs the operation, and blood transfusions are often needed. Blood transfusions are usually not required for smaller, localized tumors.

Though nephrectomy is the most common treatment for kidney cancer, it is important to note that in some cases it may not be appropriate for your situation. Your doctor will explain the factors that influence the decision on whether to proceed with a nephrectomy.

For patients who have locally advanced or metastatic disease, clinical trials are ongoing to determine the benefit of neoadjuvant therapies (therapy given for a specific time prior to surgery). The goal of these trials is to evaluate if the size of the tumor or overall disease burden can be reduced prior to surgery and perhaps allow a lesser invasive surgery, improve the surgical outcome, or improve survival. Your doctor will discuss this with you if you are eligible to participate in any available trials at your center before your surgery.

There are two basic types of nephrectomies for kidney cancer:

Radical Nephrectomy. A radical nephrectomy involves removal of the entire kidney and the surrounding fatty tissue, and may include the adrenal gland above the kidney as well as any enlarged lymph nodes adjacent to the kidney. A radical nephrectomy is a more involved surgery, and can be done in open or minimally invasive fashion. The adrenal gland, which is located immediately above the kidney, is sometimes removed during a radical nephrectomy. It may be appropriate to leave the adrenal gland behind, however, especially when the tumor is relatively small or located away from the adrenal. Partial or complete removal of the lymph nodes during surgery also may be helpful to determine if the tumor has spread, but this decision depends on a variety of factors. A pathologist will examine all the removed tissues, including the lymph nodes and the adrenal gland under a microscope to see if any kidney cancer cells are present in these tissues.

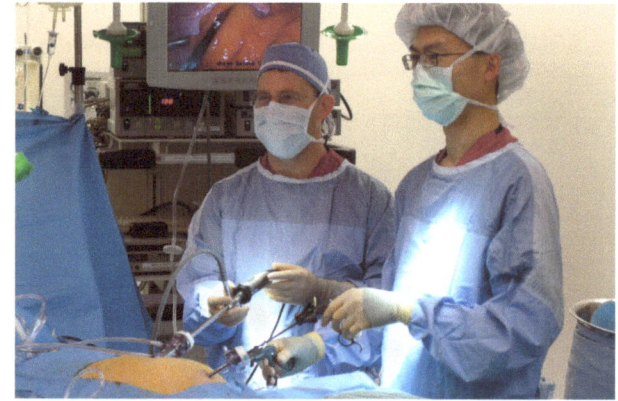

"Minimally invasive" procedures, such as laparoscopic surgery, above, can result in shorter hospital stays and recovery time.

Partial Nephrectomy. Partial nephrectomy can often achieve the same results in patients with small to medium-sized cancers. In an open partial nephrectomy, the surgeon removes just the part of the kidney that contains the tumor. Partial nephrectomy is particularly indicated in patients with small unilateral tumors, or patients having one kidney, kidney failure or familial RCC. The size and location of the tumor can also determine whether a partial nephrectomy is performed.

Partial nephrectomy can be performed using an open incision or minimally invasively using laparoscopy or robotic assistance. Partial nephrectomies are more technically challenging than a radical nephrectomy, and may not be performed by every surgeon and at every institution. You should seek a surgeon who has substantial experience and performs many partial nephrectomy procedures. At academic and other medical centers where many patients with kidney cancer are seen and more resources are available, partial nephrectomies may outnumber radical nephrectomies.

Minimally Invasive Surgeries

Less invasive surgical techniques have been developed and are widely used to perform nephrectomy and partial nephrectomy. These are now referred to as "minimally invasive surgeries," and involve the use of a laparoscope, an instrument that is passed through a series of small incisions or "ports" in the abdominal wall. Laparoscopy can be used for both radical and partial nephrectomies and accomplishes the same things as traditional surgical techniques.

The known benefits of these minimally invasive procedures include decreased blood loss, a shorter hospital stay, less need for narcotic pain medication and shorter recovery time when compared with open radical or open partial nephrectomies.

Most medical centers and many surgeons offer laparoscopic radical nephrectomy, however the use of laparoscopic instrumentation alone can be technically difficult. Hand-assisted laparoscopic nephrectomy was developed as an aid to laparoscopic nephrectomy and provides the surgeon the ability to use a hand to assist. Short incisions are made in conjunction with the instrument ports in order to insert one hand to assist the laparoscopic maneuvers. Hand-assisted laparoscopy may make laparoscopic nephrectomies more widely available while maintaining the benefits of minimally invasive surgery.

Robotic Assisted Laparoscopic Partial Nephrectomy

Robotic assisted laparoscopic partial nephrectomy is a technique that has been introduced more recently to patients at various practices. The robotic instrumentation basically makes the laparoscopic procedure easier for the surgeon to perform. The surgical robot has two components – the robotics component and surgeon console. The robot has one arm that controls a laparoscopic camera and two to three arms that control miniature laparoscopic instruments that perform various functions. The surgeon sits separately at a console in the operating room, which provides a three-dimensional view of the field and controls the robotic instruments. During standard laparoscopy, considerable experience is needed to safely remove the tumor, suture the blood vessels inside the kidney, and then sew the kidney closed. Using the robot may help make laparoscopic partial nephrectomy easier to perform by the surgeon. It is important to ask your surgeon how much experience he or she has with either laparoscopic partial nephrectomy or robotic surgery.

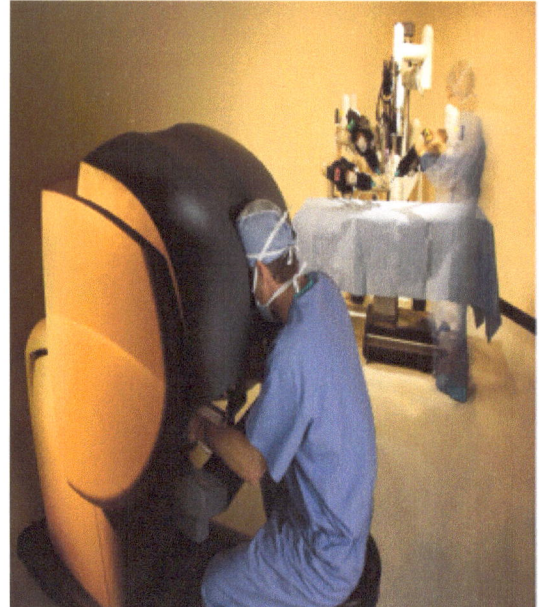

A surgeon uses a special console in robotic surgery.

Ablative Therapies

Other minimally invasive procedures, also referred to as ablative therapies, are cryoablation and radiofrequency ablation (RFA). These treatments are generally for patients who may be poor candidates for surgery. Cryosurgery, or cryoablation, uses freezing temperatures. The cryoprobe is inserted directly into the mass, either through the skin with radiologic guidance or during laparoscopic surgery. RFA is another technique used to destroy small tumors. RFA destroys tumors with thermal energy (heat).

The long-term benefits of these non-surgical ablative techniques remains to be determined, but early results for RFA are promising.

Ask your doctor what surgical technique is best for your particular case.

The Role of Nephrectomy in Advanced Disease

When cancer has spread to other parts of your body, it is referred to as metastasis.

Nephrectomy has become an integral part of the management of patients with metastatic kidney cancer. A nephrectomy may be beneficial if the cancer has already spread because your body then has less cancer to fight through treatments that your doctor might be recommending. Indications that some patients had spontaneous regression of their metastatic disease following nephrectomy, and the fact that the primary tumor rarely, if ever, responded to systemic therapy, prompted more widespread integration of nephrectomy into the management of patients with metastatic disease. Studies and data demonstrate that patients respond better to systemic therapies, particularly immunotherapies, if the kidney is removed.

A study of 241 patients with operable metastatic kidney cancer demonstrated that patients who had a nephrectomy before systemic therapy with interferon-alfa had a higher survival rate than patients treated with interferon-alfa alone.

A more recent study of 2,447 patients with metastatic kidney cancer who had a nephrectomy before systemic therapy had a higher survival rate than those who did not receive surgical intervention. Ongoing studies are reviewing survival rates for patients who receive targeted therapy and factors associated with survival of those patients.

Performing nephrectomy in patients with advanced kidney cancer is not without risk, however. Circumstances can happen which can delay or prevent starting systemic therapy after surgery. For example, metastatic disease progression can occur during the postoperative period or a complication could develop before or during surgery which may prolong recovery time. Patient selection for surgery remains critical for success. Patients should be good candidates for surgery, and have a tumor that can be safely and completely removed by surgery. Patients with complicating factors, including metastases to the liver, brain, or bones, may not be good candidates for surgery because of their poor overall prognosis.

Arterial Embolization

A procedure called arterial embolization is rarely performed, and only in special conditions. Small pieces of a special gelatin sponge or other material are injected through a catheter to block the artery that feeds the tumor-containing kidney. This procedure can shrink the tumor by depriving it of the oxygen and nutrients it needs to grow and may reduce bleeding during the operation. It is also used to provide relief from pain or bleeding when surgical removal of the tumor is not an option because of poor health or for other reasons.

How to Think About Your Tumor

Your tumor or removed tissue may be useful – both to you as a cancer patient and for cancer research in general. The tumor and other tissues that are removed surgically provide important information to your doctor about your specific cancer that may help estimate your risk of relapse and/or guide further treatments. Additionally, your tissue can contribute to research. For example, the tumor is a storehouse of white blood cells and various other constituents of the immune system that your body has recruited to fight your cancer. In some cases – always as a part of a research protocol that the patient must approve in writing prior to removing the tumor – the tissue may be used to prepare a vaccine or may be saved for other research purposes. Tissue will not be available if your tumor is destroyed by cryosurgery or RFA, and although a biopsy may have been performed before these treatments, it will not yield sufficient tissue for any other studies.

Some therapies under development use material extracted from the surgically removed tumor to fight any malignant cells left behind. It is important to note that these therapies – vaccine therapy, for example – are investigational, and results are still uncertain. Before surgery, you should discuss with your doctor what the most appropriate use of your tissue should be after it is removed. At present, however, keep in mind that there is no reason to routinely save tissue. Tissue cannot typically be saved for later therapy unless it is part of an approved research protocol offered at the institution where the surgery is to be performed. Keep in mind that these research protocols often take years to be approved by a hospital Ethics board and are heavily regulated, to the point that they cannot even be offered to the patient until the approval is in place. So if one is approved and available, keep in mind that significant effort has already been undertaken by the time you become aware of it. You should consult your doctor for a recommendation.

Before the Operation

If your doctor recommends a radical or partial nephrectomy, you will probably have lots of questions and concerns. Be sure to share these with your doctor. You will want to know where the surgery will be performed and who the surgeon will be. Your surgery should be performed in a hospital or medical center that is experienced in dealing with kidney cancer. Your surgeon should be a board-certified urologic surgeon. If you do not know whether your hospital or doctor meets these requirements, ask questions before scheduling or agreeing to surgery. No one will be offended by your prudence. You may also want to know how you will feel after the operation and how any pain you might experience will be addressed. You may want to know when you will be discharged and when you can resume normal activities and what kind of follow-up treatment is planned. Getting answers to these questions can help relieve or reduce your anxiety so you can focus on healing and fighting your cancer.

The Day Before Surgery

Prior to your surgery some simple final tests will be performed, usually when you see the anesthesiologist so he or she has information on how much anesthetic gas to give you during the operation. You may also be required to take a laxative and to drink fluids to flush out your bowels. In order to reduce the risk of infection during surgery, your surgeon does not want you to have anything in your stomach or intestines. You may also be asked to wash your body with special antibacterial soap. Clean out your belly button well. Men are advised to shave their face the night before. You may not get a chance to shave for several days after surgery. You may be a little anxious the night before surgery. You may be offered a sleeping pill to make sure you get a good night's rest before surgery. Do not shave or trim the area of surgery as this raises the risk of infection.

The Day of Surgery

Most patients report to the hospital on the day of surgery. When you arrive in the "pre-op" area on the day of surgery, the anesthesia team will prepare you for surgery. Different anesthesia techniques can be used to keep you free from pain. One common technique involves the use of an epidural catheter to administer a direct flow of anesthetic to your nervous system. This process usually starts with an injection of a local anesthetic into your back, followed by the insertion of a catheter into your back at the spine, just above your kidneys. The catheter is connected with a thin plastic tube to a pump that will give you small injections of anesthetic to prevent any pain. By administering a small, precise dose at frequent, predetermined intervals, the anesthesiologist can achieve greater safety and pain relief. With less anesthetic administered, there are few, if any, side effects. (This system is also widely used for childbirth.)

You will be transported into the operating room and the anesthesiologist will put you to sleep using a combination of anesthetic gases. The surgery will begin. You will be totally asleep and have no awareness of pain during surgery.

After the surgeon has completed the procedure and the incision is closed and bandaged, you will spend some time in a surgical recovery room. You will be carefully watched and you will slowly wake up as the effects of the anesthetic gases wear off.

You will also be very "relaxed" from the medications used to control surgical pain. Your surgeon will want you to have as little pain as possible because if you are comfortable, you will heal better. Try to relax and sleep.

If your surgery has been extensive, you may be put in an intensive care room where your recovery can be closely monitored for several days. You probably won't remember the operation or going to the recovery room. Your first recollection will probably be waking up in your hospital room or in intensive care. If you are in intensive care when you wake up, you may be surprised if you have not seen an intensive care room before. The IV bags, oxygen tubes, electronic heart monitors, and other equipment are there for only one reason – your safe recovery. Though they are distracting, they play an important role in your recovery.

In the intensive care unit, you will be closely watched by nurses and doctors. In some hospitals, you may even have nursing staff assigned exclusively to you 24 hours per day.

Your blood pressure and temperature will be checked hourly. Samples of your blood will be drawn frequently. Certain drugs may be administered to help you recover safely. If you want something or feel uncomfortable, communicate your needs to the hospital staff. They are there to help you. Depending on the hospital and your condition, you may be allowed to have visitors while you are in intensive care. Generally, visits are limited to your immediate family and only during certain hours. However, as a consequence of your medication, your visitors should not expect you to engage in much conversation. Don't expect to remember the details of your conversations while you are in the intensive care unit. It may also be upsetting for some family members to visit you in intensive care, particularly because they may not understand that all the tubes and wires are there to help you get better and that they serve a medical purpose. The best policy may be to tell the hospital staff to restrict your visitors until you are feeling better.

A Few Days After Surgery

Your recovery schedule in the two or three days after surgery will depend on what type of surgery you have had. The various tubes and other support equipment will be removed. You may be allowed to have more visitors. You will be able to read, listen to music, watch television, and take telephone calls.

Your doctors will visit regularly to check your medical condition. Medical staff will check your incision and change the bandage.

As you recover, the way you are given pain medication will change, and the epidural catheter in your back will be removed. Milder pain medications may be given by intravenous injection and/or orally. A PCA (patient controlled analgesia) pump provides small, continuous doses of pain medication that you can give yourself when you need them. This is attached to your IV line, and is typically given after open operations. Some of these medications, particularly narcotic pain relievers, may cause constipation. If so, mention this problem to your doctor. He or she may decide to switch your medication or give you something to relieve your constipation.

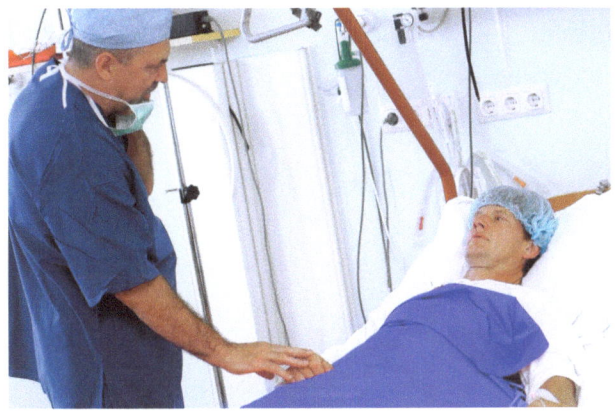

During the first few days after your surgery, the medical team will provide more information about your pathology tests, which will determine the type of tumor, whether it has spread and other important facts.

You will use an incentive spirometer (small device to assist in breathing exercises) to prevent pneumonia. You will also be instructed to do breathing and coughing exercises several times a day, to prevent lung infections. You will wear TED hose (elastic compression stockings) on your legs to improve circulation and prevent blood clots. You will wear these while you are in bed.

Exercise is an important part of recovery. It improves your circulation and respiration, and helps prevent blood clots in your legs. The day after surgery, you will be asked to get out of bed and perhaps do some walking. Getting out of bed may not be easy at first, although walking or shuffling along may be no problem. Getting into and out of bed is difficult because during an open partial or radical nephrectomy, the surgeon may need to cut through your flank muscles. He or she may also have removed one or more of your ribs. Despite any discomfort, get out of bed and walk. It's good for you. Note that if you have had a laparoscopic procedure, your recovery time may be shorter following surgery. Generally, it may be possible for laparoscopic patients to be discharged earlier. Your surgeon will be asking you if you are passing flatus (gas), as this is the most reliable sign that your gastrointestinal system has 'awakened' and is working well.

When your gastrointestinal system is ready, you will get some solid food to eat. Take care to eat well, but try to eat frequent (six or so) small meals rather than three big meals. Your body will be rebuilding muscles and other tissues. Good nourishment will help the healing process.

Going Home

If you had an open surgical procedure, about one week – or even less – after surgery, the surgical staples or sutures will be removed from your incision. This removal does not hurt. The incision will be lightly bandaged. You will be discharged and sent home to recover. You will still be taking medications to relieve pain and a prescription sleeping medication to help you sleep at night. You will still find it difficult to get into and out of bed by yourself because your back muscles are still healing. You may find it more comfortable to sit in a soft chair or even sleep in a chair, preferably one with strong arms so you can help yourself into and out of it.

It is a good idea to get some walking exercise every day. You won't be able to do any physical work or lift much weight. Take advantage of this time to relax. There isn't much you can do to speed up the healing process, so don't aggravate yourself. One word of caution – a real belly laugh can hurt, so be careful of funny movies and excessive humor. Sneezing and coughing can be painful, too.

Depending on the type of dressing used to bandage the incision, you may be able to take a shower. If a shower is not possible, take regular sponge baths. Try to take good care of yourself. It will make you feel better.

Your surgeon may want you to visit his or her office within a month after hospital discharge. The purpose of this visit is to check the healing of your incision, follow up for complications, conduct blood and urine tests, and check your health after surgery. It is also a time for your doctor to share with you the final results from the pathology report and discuss with you follow-up oncological care. If you are having any problems or feel something isn't going right, be sure to discuss these concerns with your doctor.

Depending upon your type of work activity and the type of operation (open or minimally invasive), your surgeon will advise you when you may return to work and can provide a return to work letter. Some people may return to work as soon as two weeks after surgery if they are feeling well, but they typically return in four to six weeks. During this recovery period, it is important to pace yourself because it can take a full three months for your muscles to heal and to regain your strength.

About two months after your surgery, you can start doing more exercises. Build up to the level of exercise that effectively works different muscles but is still comfortable for you. Exercise will help restore your muscle tone and your energy level.

The recovery process described above is typical for open radical nephrectomies. Recovery times may be considerably shorter after a partial nephrectomy or laparoscopic procedures. For ablative procedures, your hospital stay will probably be an overnight stay, and your recovery shorter than the other procedures. It is always a good idea to ask your doctor's advice before resuming exercise after surgery. Your doctor may have instructions which are different from other doctors – and which may also depend upon the extent of your surgery.

Prognosis

The tumor and kidney removed will be examined by trained experts called pathologists. During the first days or weeks following surgery, they perform detailed analyses of the removed tissues. Details may include the type of tumor, whether the tumor has spread to the lymph nodes or other surrounding organs, and other facts that are important for you to know, since these will impact your prognosis. Your surgeon should discuss the results of these tests, called the Pathology Report, with you and translate it as it usually contains a lot of medical jargon. You should feel comfortable asking questions about the report, including the type (histology), stage and grade of your tumor.

The good news is that survival rates for kidney cancer have improved, as they have for many types of cancer. The probability of long-term survival depends on a combination of factors, particularly the spread of the tumor as defined by stage.

About half of all patients have localized disease (Stage I or II) and have an excellent prognosis for long-term survival.

In addition to the TNM stage of your tumor, survival is affected by its grade level. Grade – also known as "Fuhrman grade" for RCC patients – is different than stage, and is determined by the pathologist who examines the tissue. The grade refers to how closely the cancer cells look like normal kidney cells. Tumor grade is defined by the size and density of cancer cell nuclei, as judged by pathologic microscopic evaluation. Renal cell cancers are graded on a scale of 1 through 4.

Grade 1 cells are most like normal cells and are thus less aggressive. They often grow slowly, and patients with grade 1 cells generally have a good prognosis. At the other extreme, grade 4 cells are very different from normal cells. They are more likely to be invasive and more likely to metastasize. More information about the grading and staging of kidney cancer can be found in Chapter 2 of this book.

As tumor spread (stage) increases, so does the probability of lymph node involvement and the chance that malignant cells may have microscopically spread to other parts of the body.

Despite the statistical research on survival, be careful not to generalize from average survival summaries to your own case. Survival statistics vary from study to study. Many survival studies have used small samples so the results may not be applicable to larger patient populations. Moreover, no kidney cancer case is average. Every case is unique. These facts cannot be emphasized too much, to you, the patient.

Your probability of long-term survival will also depend on your age and physical condition, the type of follow-up and treatment received after your nephrectomy, and a host of other tumor-related factors. You should discuss your survival prognosis with your doctor, because he or she is most familiar with the unique medical characteristics of your case. Don't be surprised if your doctor is reluctant to give you an exact answer, however, because he or she is aware of the many variables that can affect survival and knows there is no precise answer.

You should also keep this last thought in mind: the longer you survive, with or without disease, the better your chances of receiving a new, more effective treatment. Significant advances have been made in the past two decades and much exciting research is being done at this very moment. The longer the time goes from your initial treatment, the more benefit you may get from this clinical research.

Medical Follow-Up

After nephrectomy, you should have frequent medical check-ups. How often and what tests are scheduled will be determined by your doctor based on your situation at the time of diagnosis, the pathology of your particular tumor, and other factors. Your doctor may schedule regular diagnostic tests. If after a period of several years no more cancer is evident, your doctor may decide to reduce the frequency of these tests or transition you to Survivorship care.

Just as the stage of your cancer (I, II, III, or IV) helps determine the treatment options considered by your health care team, it also affects the follow-up care you will receive following your initial treatment.

In general, the higher your stage of cancer at the time of initial treatment, the more intensive and frequent your follow-up care will be. For example, the frequency of doctor visits will be higher for Stage III patients than for Stage I patients. Follow-up procedures may also be more intense; for example, a simple chest x-ray may suffice as a check-up for early-stage patients, but a CT scan may be necessary for later-stage patients.

Stage I and Stage II patients receive no other treatment than close follow-up care. Even for Stage III patients, the standard is no additional treatment. However, patients with Stage III disease may be treated with more aggressive follow-up that includes some form of additional treatment (known as adjuvant therapy), currently in the context of a clinical trial. Patients with Stage IV disease (cancer that has spread to other organs) almost always receive treatment and this includes some form of additional regularly scheduled follow-up.

During your follow-up period, you should watch for the unique signs and symptoms that occurred when you first noticed the disease. For some people, certain symptoms or blood test abnormalities may be useful indicators of recurrent disease.

You should also keep a journal of your aches and pains and any other physical ailments you experience. Bring your journal to your check-ups. If you experience any unusual pains or symptoms between check-ups, call your doctor. If something is wrong, you will get help sooner. If nothing is wrong, you will have peace of mind after talking to your doctor. Even if your prognosis is excellent, you and your doctor should be vigilant. If any metastases occur, you want to catch the problem early and treat it promptly because immediate attention will prolong your survival.

Things to Look for Between Check-ups

Your doctor does not work alone in keeping you healthy. He or she relies on you to discuss any problems you have. If you experience any of the following problems, be sure to call them to your doctor's attention: weight loss, loss of appetite, weakness, headache, changes in your mental status, recurrent fevers or high temperature, abdominal or skeletal pain, a cough that does not go away, shortness of breath, enlarged lymph glands, or blood in your urine. Be careful. Do not dismiss symptoms of illness as unimportant. Your doctor will not criticize you for being cautious.

Treatment Considerations

If there is no evidence of metastases after your nephrectomy, your doctor may decide, based on current medical information, that no additional treatment is necessary beyond medical check-ups. However, if you do fall into the category of "high-risk" recurrence, you might benefit from additional treatment – known as adjuvant therapy – treatment given after your nephrectomy (more about this is described in the next chapter). These treatments can be quite different from one another. Currently no standard adjuvant therapy is recommended as no effective agents have yet been found, but clinical trials are investigating the possible benefits of such therapy. Specific criteria must be met for a patient to be "eligible" for an adjuvant clinical trial.

Many patients ask about the use of radiation or chemotherapy as a treatment for their kidney cancer. It is important to note that typical kidney cancer is not as responsive to these therapies as other forms of cancer are; thus radiation and chemotherapy are not used as primary treatment.

More information about these treatments is included in the chapter "Therapies for Advanced Kidney Cancer."

Summary

For most kidney cancer patients, radical or partial nephrectomy will be a part of your treatment plan. This surgery is performed thousands of times every year and is quite safe and effective. New advances in surgical technique offer less-invasive forms of surgery and shorter hospital stays. If your cancer is treated by surgery early enough, complications are few and prognosis may be good. For patients with more advanced-stage cancer, additional treatment may be required; still, for many of these patients, surgery plays an important role.

NOTES

Oral drugs offer many benefits as a treatment

"I was diagnosed with kidney cancer on New Year's Day, 2004. I thought I had been having a kidney-stone attack, which we have a history of in my family. But an x ray showed a large tumor in my only kidney. I had a partial nephrectomy and went on with my life.

But in December of that year, another x ray turned up an enlargement in the lymph nodes behind my aorta. They told me the cancer had spread. That was quite an emotional setback. I was told that I probably had about 6 months to live. But my urologist suggested I did have an option – to participate in a research trial with experimental oral drugs at a clinic in another state. So I applied for the program.

I'll never forget the day I went in to the clinic to find out if I would be eligible for the trial, Valentines Day. When the nurse came out, smiled and handed me the pills I was to take as a part of the trial, it was a great moment. I've had a lot of highs and lows since being diagnosed, but that was one of the real high points for me.

I started taking the oral treatment in February of 2005 and within six months two of the tumors were gone and the largest lymph node involved had shrunk to its original size. I'm still taking the medication from the clinical trial, which has since been approved and is now available as a prescription, and have been free of tumors.

Just like any medication, there are some side effects. I have had some discomfort in my hands and feet – it's easy to form blisters. And occasionally I have some nausea. But over time I have adjusted. You learn which foods you can eat and which you should avoid, and there are other things you can do to help the side effects. I sometimes wear gloves when I'm doing certain things, for example, to help prevent blisters. The side effects change your lifestyle a little bit, but it's not bad. I really appreciate being able to take the medication at home rather than getting treated at a hospital. It's literally been a life saver for me.

The key, I think, in fighting kidney cancer is: don't let it stop you. Keep planning and living your life, pushing yourself to stay active at any level you can. Focus on the life you have right now. Stay positive and enjoy every day you are given. I am better off today than before I had cancer. I know what is important in life and I am a better person for the experience."

CHAPTER 4

THERAPIES FOR ADVANCED KIDNEY CANCER

The treatment for your kidney cancer may not involve surgery alone. A number of other systemic therapies are available that can be highly successful.

Sometimes surgical treatment alone is not sufficient for kidney cancer. If you had metastatic disease (cancer that has spread to other organs) when you were diagnosed, or if you have developed metastatic cancer since your nephrectomy, your doctor will most likely recommend additional treatment. The most commonly used treatments for kidney cancer are various forms of "targeted therapies" or immunotherapy. Targeted therapies – so-called because they "target" cancer at the cellular level – have expanded the options for the treatment of kidney cancer.

Other traditional – but less-often used – treatments include radiation therapy and chemotherapy. Several investigational therapies, including vaccine therapy, are also available.

Targeted Therapy

One of the most exciting new developments in recent years has been the introduction of drugs that interfere with the growth of cancer cells at a molecular level. By focusing on specific molecular growth pathways, these drugs can interfere with cell growth, prevent cell replication, or disrupt the blood flow supply to the cell.

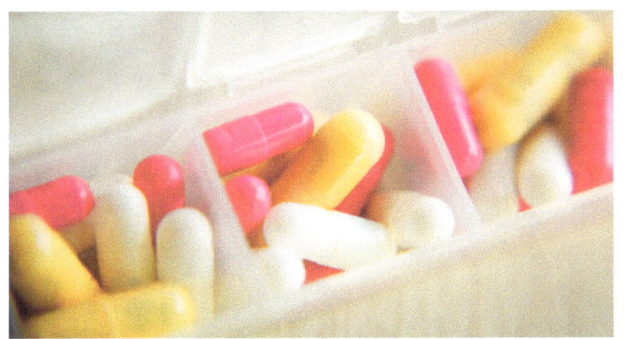

The introduction of drugs in recent years that interfere with the growth of kidney cancer cells has given a new sense of hope for patients.

Much research is under way worldwide and it is yielding new targeted therapies as well as providing information about how they work. As more is learned about pathways of cells, it is likely that even more new drugs and treatments will be introduced.

Angiogenesis Inhibitors

For malignant tumors to grow and metastasize, they must be able to form new blood vessels by a process called angiogenesis.

Tumors overproduce "growth factors" that stimulate the development of new blood vessels to supply oxygen and nutrition. These include "vascular endothelial growth factor" (VEGF) and "platelet-derived growth factor" (PDGF). These growth factors activate certain tyrosine kinases, proteins inside cancer cells that are important in cell functions, including the development of new blood vessels. This allows tumors to grow and to metastasize to other parts of the body.

In 2005 and 2006, the U.S. Food and Drug Administration (FDA) approved the first new medications to treat kidney cancer in more than a decade: Nexavar® (sorafenib tosylate) and Sutent® (sunitinib malate). Both of these drugs disrupt the angiogenesis process. In 2009, the FDA approved two additional angiogenesis inhibitors called Votrient® (pazopanib) and Avastin® (bevacizumab), given in combination with Intron (interferon). In 2012, it approved a similar drug called Inlyta® (axitinib), and in 2016 it approved a drug called Cabometyx®(cabozantinib).

Sorafenib, sunitinib, pazopanib, axitinib, lenvatinib, and cabozantinib are known as tyrosine kinase inhibitors, or TKIs. These medications interfere with the proteins inside cancer cells, thus interfering with certain cell functions. All six of these drugs are administered orally, and show great promise for kidney cancer patients. These drugs are also known as "multi-kinase inhibitors" because they target both the tumor cell and the tumor blood vessel structures. They work by interfering with reproduction of cancer cells as they attempt to grow and divide uncontrollably. Axitinib is also a TKI that is used to treat advanced kidney cancer in patients when one prior drug treatment is no longer effective in controlling the disease. Cabozantinib differs in that it targets multiple tyrosine kinases involved in the development of kidney cancer.

The goal of treatment with these medications is to slow the rate of growth of the cancer and, if possible, shrink the size of existing tumors. Some patients may experience a significant decrease in the amount of cancer in their body. Some patients may not experience shrinkage in the size of their tumors, but have long periods of "stable" disease. (See section titled "Managing Your Expectations of Therapy" later in this chapter). Ongoing research efforts are pursuing additional medications that will be effective in treating kidney cancer (see chapter six, "Clinical Trials"). Your physician will discuss how your cancer is responding to treatment, and will have additional options to consider for treatment when necessary.

It should be noted that some patients will not receive any benefit from a medication. In some cases, a medication that was effective in treating a patient's cancer stops working and other treatment options must be considered.

Certain foods, medications, and complimentary therapies will affect the absorption of oral medications. Therefore it is important for patients to inform their physicians and dentists about the medications, vitamins, and complimentary therapies they are taking. Medications can be changed to avoid decreasing the effectiveness or increasing the side effects associated with medication interactions.

Your oncologist, nurse practitioner, physician assistant, or oncology nurse will give you more detailed information regarding possible side effects of treatment, and the type and frequency of blood tests to monitor how you're doing with treatment. They will also tell you how often CT scans, MRI scans, or bone scans will be done to determine how effective treatment is.

Nexavar® (sorafenib tosylate)

Nexavar® (sorafenib tosylate) is a medication that targets the blood supply of a tumor, depriving it of the oxygen and nutrients it needs for growth. By blocking the vascular endothelial growth factor (VEGF) and platelet-derived growth factor (PDGF), Nexavar® can interfere with the tumor cell's ability to increase its blood supply. By blocking the Raf-kinase pathway, Nexavar® can also interfere with tumor cell growth and proliferation. Clinical studies show that it can significantly slow the progression of tumors. In the Phase III trial which led to the FDA approval of Nexavar®, the median time for tumor progression was doubled for patients taking Nexavar®, compared with patients taking a placebo.

Nexavar® is available as a 200mg tablet. The approved dose of Nexavar® is 400mg (two 200mg tablets) taken twice a day, approximately 12 hours apart. Because food will affect the absorption of Nexavar®, it is important to take this medication one hour before or two hours after eating. Nexavar® is taken every day in a continuous fashion, with four weeks of dosing typically considered to be a "cycle" of treatment. Certain medications and complimentary therapies will affect the absorption of Nexavar®, therefore it is important for patients to inform their physicians and dentists about the medications, vitamins, and complimentary therapies they are taking. Medications can be changed to avoid decreasing the effectiveness or increasing the side effects associated with Nexavar® due to medication interactions.

Some of the common side effects of Nexavar® include fatigue, diarrhea, rash or redness of the skin, itching, high blood pressure, hand-foot-skin-reaction (pain, redness, calluses, or peeling of the skin), hair loss, mouth irritation, decreased appetite, and low blood phosphorus level. For additional information visit www.nexavar.com.

Sutent® (sunitinib malate)

Sutent® (sunitinib malate) deprives tumor cells of the blood and nutrients needed to grow by interfering with VEGF and PDGF signaling pathways. Sutent® was initially approved by the FDA in 2006 for kidney cancer patients because of its ability to reduce the size of tumors. Clinical studies showed a favorable response rate in patients with metastatic kidney cancer whose tumors had progressed following immunotherapy. Sutent® received full approval for the treatment of advanced renal cell carcinoma in February 2007 based on data from the first line study of Sutent® versus Interferon in patients with metastatic renal cancer who had not received prior treatment.

Sutent® is available in several different capsule strengths (50 mg, 25 mg, and 12.5 mg). Your doctor will prescribe the appropriate capsule strength according to your daily dose. The approved dose for starting treatment with Sutent® is 50mg daily taken once a day for 28 days, followed by a 14-day rest (no Sutent® to be taken). A "cycle" of treatment with Sutent® is considered a 6-week period, 28 days of Sutent and a 14-day rest. This is considered an "intermittent dosing schedule." The dose of Sutent® can be adjusted based on side effects a patient experiences during treatment. Because certain other medications and complementary therapies will affect the absorption of Sutent®, it is very important for patients to inform their physicians and dentists about the medications, vitamins, and complimentary therapies they are taking. Medications can be changed to avoid decreasing the effectiveness or increasing the side effects associated with Sutent® due to medication interactions.

Some of the common side effects of Sutent® include fatigue, diarrhea, nausea, mouth irritation, taste changes, decreased appetite, high blood pressure, hand-foot-syndrome (pain, redness, calluses, or peeling of the skin), hypothyroidism, and low blood counts (white blood cells, neutrophils, platelets). For more information about Sutent®, please visit www.sutent.com.

Votrient® (pazopanib)

Votrient® (pazopanib) was approved in October 2009 for the treatment of advanced kidney cancer. Like Sutent and Nexavar, it deprives tumor cells of the blood and nutrients needed to grow. Clinical studies showed a favorable response rate in patients with metastatic kidney cancer. Votrient® is an oral medication, and the recommended starting dose is 800mg once daily without food (at least 1 hour before or 2 hours after a meal). Your oncologist may recommend that you temporarily interrupt your treatment and/or reduce your dose of Votrient® if you develop severe side effects. Patients with reduced liver function should start at 200 mg once daily. Your doctor will make this recommendation for you if it is appropriate.

Some of the common side effects of Votrient® include fatigue, diarrhea, high blood pressure, nausea, vomiting, abdominal pain, mouth irritation, decreased appetite, and abnormal liver function tests (AST, ALT, bilirubin). For more information about Votrient®, please visit www.votrient.com.

Inlyta® (axitinib)

Inlyta® (axitinib) is a medication used to treat advanced kidney cancer in adults when one prior drug treatment is no longer effective in controlling the disease. It was approved by the U.S. Food and Drug Administration in January 2012 based on a Phase III study which showed that axitinib provided significant benefit for patients when compared to sorafenib following "front-line" treatment. Inlyta® works by blocking proteins called kinases, which play an important role in the growth of tumors and the progression of cancer, and is similar to sunitinib, sorafenib, and pazopanib. Inlyta® is an oral medication which comes in 5 mg and 1 mg tablets, and is taken twice a day, approximately 12 hours apart. It can be taken with or without food.

Some of the common side effects of Inlyta® include fatigue, diarrhea, high blood pressure, nausea, mouth irritation, decreased appetite, hand-foot-syndrome, voice changes, hypothyroidism, and proteinuria. For more information about Inlyta®, please visit www.inlyta.com.

Cabometyx® (cabozantinib)

Cabometyx® (cabozantinib) was approved in April 2016 for the treatment of advanced kidney cancer following treatment with an anti-antigenic therapy. If you are contemplating an elective surgical procedure, stop treatment with Cabometyx® for at least 28 days prior to the scheduled surgery. This includes dental surgery.

In a Phase III randomized clinical study that compared Cabometyx® to Afinitor®, patients with previously treated advanced kidney cancer that received treatment with Cabometyx® lived longer, had a longer progression-free survival and a greater objective response rate. Cabometyx® differs from other approved treatment options, as it targets multiple tyrosine kinases involved in the development of RCC, including MET, AXL and three VEGF receptors. MET, AXL and VEGF receptors are proteins found on the surface of cancer cells that can pro-mote tumor angiogenesis (blood vessel growth), growth, inva-siveness and metastasis. Cabometyx® works by targeting these receptors and can decrease the growth of new blood vessels to tumors and the spread of cancer cells, while inhibiting drug resistance.

Cabometyx® is a tablet that is taken daily at the same time each day. It comes in three strengths, 20 mg, 40 mg, and 60 mg. The starting dose is 60 mg daily, and should not be taken with food. The tablets are not scored and therefore cannot be cut in half. Health care teams today are familiar with this class of drug and have experience with how to manage dosages in order to maintain balance safety and efficacy.

Some of the common side effects of Cabometyx® include fatigue, diarrhea, high blood pressure, nausea, mouth irritation, decreased appetite, hand-foot-syndrome, abnormal liver func-tion tests (AST, ALT), increased creatinine, and increased triglycerides. For more information about Cabometyx®, please visit https://hcp.cabometyx.com.

Lenvima® (lenvatinib) + Afinitor® (everolimus)

On May 13, 2016, the FDA approved the first ever two-drug combination for the treatment of advanced kidney cancer. The treatment is indicated in patients who have been previously treated with anti-angiogenic therapy.

Approval of the drug combination was based on a Phase II randomized multi-center study with the objective of improving progression-free survival in patients. Patients who were given Lenvima® and Afinitor® in combination were found to have an improved progression-free survival compared to patients treated with Lenvima® alone or Afinitor® alone. In other words, the combination of Lenvima® and Afinitor® remained effective for a longer period of time than each drug given as a single agent. Each drug targets a different mechanism of cancer growth. Lenvima® targets blood vessel formation and Afinitor® targets cancer cell growth by interrupting the availability of nutrients.

The recommended dose for Lenvima® is 18 mg (one 10 mg tablet and two 4 mg tablets) taken with a 5 mg tablet of Afinitor® on a daily basis. Both drugs should be taken together at the same time every day, with or without food. Foods to avoid while taking these medications are grapefruit, grapefruit juice and star fruit. The tablets should not be crushed and should be stored in a cool, dry place.

Some of the common side effects of Lenvima® include fatigue, diarrhea, high blood pressure, nausea, vomiting, mouth irritation, decreased appetite, muscle or joint pain, swelling of the legs, and hypothyroidism. For more information about Lenvima®, please visit www.lenvima.com.

Your health care team is familiar with these medications and has experience in managing any side effects that may occur. Please report any side effects promptly.

For additional information regarding Lenvima® and Afinitor® in combination, please visit www.lenvima.com/advanced-kidney-cancer.

mTOR Inhibitors

The mammalian Target of rapamycin (mTOR) is an enzyme involved in regulating cellular response to nutrients and growth factors. mTOR is one of the main regulators of cell growth and proliferation. There are multiple pathways in which mTOR is regulated. In different cancers the signaling pathways that activate mTOR are altered and affecting tumor growth. Two mTOR inhibitors used in RCC are Torisel® (temsirolimus) and Afinitor® (everolimus).

Torisel® (temsirolimus)

Torisel® (temsirolimus) is a medication for the treatment of patients with advanced kidney cancer. Torisel® specifically inhibits the mTOR (mammalian target of rapamycin) kinase, a key protein in cells that regulates cell proliferation, cell growth and cell survival. In a three-arm, phase III clinical trial of 626 patients with advanced kidney cancer and poor prognostic factors who had received no prior systemic therapy, Torisel® significantly increased median overall survival compared to interferon alpha. Torisel® was FDA-approved based on the results of this study. The drug is administered as a weekly IV infusion.

Some of the common side effects of Torisel® include rash, fatigue, mouth irritation, nausea, decreased appetite, swelling of the legs, low blood counts (hemoglobin, platelets), increased blood sugar, increased cholesterol, and increased triglycerides. For more information about Torisel®, please visit www.wyeth.com/hcp/torisel/resources/patient.

Afinitor® (everolimus)

Afinitor® (everolimus) is an oral mTOR inhibitor approved for patients with advanced kidney cancer based on a phase III study in patients whose disease had worsened during treatment with sunitinib, sorafenib, bevacizumab, interleukin-2, or interferon. The clinical trial showed that Afinitor® can delay the growth or spread of kidney cancer compared to patients who did not receive Afinitor®.

Afinitor® is administered orally, as a tablet. The recommended dose of Afinitor® is 10 mg, to be taken once daily at the same time every day. Afinitor® should be kept in the original package until it is time to take your dose in order to protect it from light and moisture, and should never be chewed or crushed. The dose for Afinitor® may be decreased to 5 mg daily due to severe side effects.

Some of the common side effects of Afinitor® include mouth irritation, infections, rash, fatigue, diarrhea, swelling of the legs, nausea, decreased appetite, decreased blood counts (hemoglobin, white blood cells, platelets), and increased triglycerides.

The use of live vaccines and close contact with those who have received live vaccines should be avoided during treatment with Afinitor®.

For more information about Afinitor®, please visit www.afinitor.com/index.jsp.

Monoclonal Antibodies

An antibody is a protein produced by the body's immune system that fights infections and foreign substances in the body.

Monoclonal antibodies are genetically engineered antibodies that are identical copies of one another. They are used in various medical diagnostic tests and are being studied actively for possible use in the treatment of metastatic kidney cancer. Monoclonal antibodies can be designed to attach to particular sites on a tumor and may be used to produce images for diagnostic purposes or to deliver anti-cancer drugs to the tumor with great specificity.

Avastin® (bevacizumab)

Avastin® (bevacizumab) is FDA-approved for both colon cancer and kidney cancer, as well as breast cancer, lung cancer and glioma.

It has been investigated in a variety of clinical trials. Avastin® targets the VEGF molecule in the bloodstream and prevents VEGF from stimulating new blood-vessel formation. Several clinical trials have demonstrated the potential benefit for Avastin® in combination with interferon alfa in treating kidney cancer. (To learn more about interferons, see the section titled "Interferons" below.) Several clinical trials have been completed showing that patients who received Avastin® plus interferon alfa had control or improvement in their disease compared to those who received interferon alfa alone.

Some of the common side effects of Avastin® include nose-bleeds, fatigue, headache, high blood pressure, taste changes, decreased appetite, runny nose, dry skin, and proteinuria. For more information about Avastin®, please visit www.avastin.com.

Immunotherapy

Your body's immune system is responsible for protecting you from viruses, bacteria, and cancer cells. Immunotherapy, sometimes called biologic therapy, or biotherapy, is a form of treatment that boosts the body's own immune defenses. Immunotherapy is considered one of the standard treatment options for kidney cancer patients with advanced metastatic disease.

Well-documented, but very rare, cases of spontaneous regressions in kidney cancer patients with metastatic disease suggest that the immune system can play an important role in the control and potential treatment of this disease.

The building blocks of immunotherapy are biologic response-modifiers (BRMs). They are substances that enhance the body's immune system and improve its ability to fight cancer. BRMs do their work by regulating the intensity and duration of immune responses. A BRM can be either a manmade drug or a natural substance produced by the body.

Several BRMs can boost the body's natural immune defenses. The cytokines are an important family of BRMs that include Interleukin-2 (IL-2) and Interferons. Used either alone or in combination, they have represented the standard in the treatment of kidney cancer.

For more information regarding Interleukin-2, visit https://www.proleukin.com.

Interleukin-2

Interleukin-2 is used in the treatment of advanced kidney cancer. It stimulates the growth of two types of white blood cells: T cells and "natural killer" (NK) cells. T cells are very important in your body's fight against cancer because they recognize cancer cells and set off an alarm to the body. The NK cells respond to this alarm and are transformed into lymphokine-activated killer (LAK) cells, which are capable of destroying cancer cells.

Interleukin-2 was approved by the FDA in 1992 for the treatment of metastatic renal cell carcinoma. A genetically engineered product, recombinant IL-2, is sold under the name Proleukin® and is manufactured by Prometheus Laboratories Inc. It is available for use in various therapeutic regimens.

Several different routes of administration may be used: IV bolus, subcutaneous (SC), and continuous IV infusion (CIV). These are further classified as high-dose (IV bolus) or low-dose (SC and CIV). The term "high-dose or IV bolus" refers to the relatively large dose of the drug (IL-2) given intravenously as a 15-minute infusion every 8 hours for a maximum of 14 infusions to hasten or magnify a therapeutic response. When administered in this fashion, patients are admitted to the hospital for the duration of the treatment cycle and are closely monitored.

Recent statistics on long-term survival in patients treated with high-dose IL-2 continue to demonstrate that this therapy is effective for selected patients with metastatic renal cell carcinoma. Studies are determining which patients benefit most.

These results confirm the premise that immunotherapy has curative potential in metastatic renal cell carcinoma. In some cases, IL-2 therapy produces what are known as "durable complete responses" (results lasting greater than 10 years) in a small percentage of treated patients, representing a significant milestone in the treatment of kidney cancer.

Significant toxicities are associated with IL-2 treatment. Side effects include nausea, vomiting, hypotension, kidney dysfunction, cardiac arrythmias, diarrhea, loss of appetite, gastrointestinal bleeding, rashes, disorientation, hallucinations, fever, and chills. Most of these side effects are completely reversible on discontinuation of drug administration, but they can be severe. It is imperative that the treating doctor be experienced in the use of IL-2 and ensures diligent clinical monitoring of the patient during treatment.

For more information regarding Interleukin-2, visit https://www.proleukin.com.

Interferons

Interferons have been widely used to treat kidney cancer, alone or in combination with other drugs. Interferon therapy is typically self-administered by injection under the skin several times per week. Interferons work by "interfering" with the life processes within the cancer cell, preventing its growth and making the cell more susceptible to attack by other elements of the immune system.

There are three major types of interferons – **alfa**, **beta**, and **gamma** – but interferon alfa has been most widely studied in the treatment of kidney cancer. Several interferon alfa products are available in the United States and have been used in the treatment of kidney cancer. INTRON® A, a product of Schering Corporation has been designated as interferon alfa-2b.

In several dozen clinical trials, an overall response rate of about 13% has been achieved with interferon alfa. It is also recognized that patients who receive interferon alpha, when compared with those who are treated with hormones or chemotherapy, have improved survival rates. Response to interferon alfa is characterized by slow regression of tumors; the average time from start of treatment to shrinkage of the tumor is three to four months.

Some of the common side effects of interferon therapy include fever, chills, muscle aches, headache, decreased appetite, fatigue, depression, heart rhythm changes (arrhythmias), and low white blood count. If severe, side effects may require stopping the therapy. Fortunately, the side effects of interferon are not permanent. A dose of 5 to 20 million units of interferon alfa daily appeared to have maximal efficacy and avoided the more serious toxicities associated with higher doses. Today, interferon is recommended at a lower dose, however, and more intermittent dosing is used with similar efficacy and better tolerance.

For more information about interferon, please visit www.merckaccessprogram.com/hcp/intron-a/ or www.chemocare.com/chemotherapy/drug-info/interferon-alfa.aspx.

Immune checkpoint inhibitors (anti PD-1 and anti-PDL-1 immunotherapy)

Immune checkpoint inhibitors are exciting new treatments that show great promise in treating cancer. Immune checkpoint pathways are used to communicate between tumor cells and immune cells called T-cells, using molecules on the surface of cells. Some cancer cells have proteins on their cell surfaces that can shut off the immune response, which puts the brakes on T-cells' ability to attack cancer cells. Immune checkpoint inhibitors are medications that block cancer cells from being able to turn on the brakes, and lets the immune cell response continue. Immune checkpoint inhibitors are currently being used to fight many different forms of cancer.

Opdivo® (nivolumab)

Opdivo® is an immune checkpoint inhibitor that blocks the PD-1 checkpoint pathway. It has recently been approved by the FDA for use in the treatment of kidney cancer in patients whose kidney cancer has spread or grown after treatment with other cancer medications. It has shown the ability to extend survival in some patients. It is given by intravenous infusion over 60 minutes every two weeks. The treatment continues unless the cancer grows or if side effects become too severe.

Opdivo® sometimes causes serious side effects. It may cause your immune system to attack normal organs and tissues and affect their function. These problems may happen at any time during treatment or even be delayed until after treatment is ended. Some of the common side effects of Opdivo® include fatigue, rash, diarrhea, nausea, decreased appetite, muscle aches, joint pain, cough, anemia, and increased creatinine.

As with any cancer treatment, it is important that you tell your nurse or doctor immediately if you have any side effects after starting treatment. Not all patients experience treatment-related side effects. Talk to your oncologist for more information about this treatment and possible immune-related side effects. Discuss whether you might benefit from an immune checkpoint inhibitor, such as nivolumab. For more information about Opdivo®, please visit www.opdivotherapy.com.

Other Treatments

Radiation Therapy

Though it is not considered a primary form of therapy, radiation can be used in the treatment of kidney cancer that has metastasized to the bone, brain or spine.

Please see more detailed information about radiation therapy in Chapter 5.

Chemotherapy

Chemotherapy works on the same principles as radiation therapy except that chemicals are used to kill malignant cells or slow their growth. The specific type of chemotherapy depends on the site of metastases, type and grade of tumor, and physical condition of the patient. Many chemotherapy programs combine several different drugs to kill malignant cells that might be resistant to a single drug. Chemotherapy may be administered in a hospital or on an outpatient basis. The drugs may be taken by mouth, by intravenous infusion, or by simple injection.

Although chemotherapy is the standard treatment for most solid tumors, kidney cancer is generally resistant to chemotherapy. The reason for the resistance of kidney cancer cells to chemotherapy is not completely understood. However, it is now known that kidney cancer cells produce an overabundance of multidrug-resistance-associated protein, which acts to repel various chemotherapeutic agents away from the cancer cell.

Therefore, at present, chemotherapy is generally used in combination with other therapies or reserved for patients entering clinical trials to test new agents and for patients who failed to respond to immunotherapy. Researchers continue to study new drugs, new drug combinations, and new treatment approaches.

As in radiation therapy, chemicals can damage normal cells. As a result, patients may experience side effects such as nausea, vomiting, diarrhea, rash, allergic reactions, and low white blood cell counts. The severity of these side effects depends on dosage, the specific drug used, the patient, the course of treatment, and other factors. These effects may last for a few hours to a few days.

Investigational Therapies

Vaccine Therapy

Vaccine therapy is an experimental treatment that uses the

patient's own tumor cells or tumor-associated products to vaccinate the patient. The goal is to boost the body's immune system in order to fight cancer. Unlike other vaccines, which are preventative, cancer vaccines are therapeutic; that is, they treat the disease rather than prevent it. Once you have had surgery to remove a tumor, a portion of it is used to create a vaccine that is then re-introduced into the body. It is hoped that these naturally occurring substances will stimulate the immune system to attack any new cells that re-appear bearing the original tumor's genetic code. Vaccine therapy using tumor cells should be discussed as a treatment option before your nephrectomy, if this is planned.

Vaccine therapy is still in an investigational stage, with numerous research programs in progress. Early results were mixed, but as techniques have evolved, results have become more promising.

Adjuvant Treatments

Adjuvant trials test the effectiveness of treatments intended to reduce the risk of cancer recurrence. You may participate in a trial to test adjuvant treatment after your primary surgery. Patients who have no indication of cancer on CT scans following surgical removal of the primary kidney tumor may be candidates to participate in adjuvant clinical trials. Specific criteria must be met for a patient to be "eligible" for an adjuvant clinical trial, and these trials begin very soon after you have recovered from surgery. It is best to discuss the option of an adjuvant trial before surgery so that you do not miss possible opportunities for adjuvant treatment.

Several clinical trials have been done to determine if treating patients who are considered to be "high risk" following surgery will decrease the risk or delay the time to development of metastatic disease. Each clinical trial defines what is considered "high risk," as several factors are considered to contribute to the determination of an individual's risk of having cancer spread or metastasize. Several clinical trials have been completed, none of which have demonstrated a benefit in adjuvant treatment. Additional adjuvant trials are ongoing.

Combination/Investigational Therapies

When two drugs are put together for the first time it is considered an investigational approach. Typically, this is done in a research institution/setting on a clinical trial. These studies look for better response rates but also closely monitor side effects to ensure patient safety.

Additional investigational therapies and new drugs are being considered for efficacy with kidney cancer; these are considered phase one trials.

Stem Cell Transplants

Blood stem cells reside in the bone marrow and perform the critical role of continually replenishing the body's supply of red blood cells, white blood cells, and platelets. When transplanted, stem cells and T-Lymphocytes can elicit an anti-tumor effect under certain conditions.

This is a highly experimental procedure, and patients with advanced metastatic cancer who did not respond to standard therapy have been treated with transplantation of peripheral blood stem cells. The results of this approach remain experimental. The side effects experienced by some patients can be serious, and further refinement of the procedure and selection of patients is needed. Check with your doctor.

Managing Your Expectations of Therapy

As you and your medical team consider options, including all of the treatment therapies listed here, it's important to keep all of these options in perspective. Your doctor will make a recommendation to you based on a number of factors. It is important to understand why a particular treatment is chosen, so be sure to ask questions.

The status of your disease will be followed through the use of scheduled CT scans. Your doctor will discuss your results with you, indicating whether the tests show stabilization (known as "stable disease"), partial response, complete response, or progression of the disease.

Here are definitions of these terms:

Complete Response: Disappearance of all tumors.

Partial Response: At least a 30 percent decrease in the size of tumors.

Progressive Disease: At least a 20 percent increase in the size of tumors, or the apperance of new tumors.

Stable Disease: Shrinkage of tumors is not sufficient to qualify for a partial response nor is there sufficient growth of tumors to qualify for progressive disease.

Your doctor measures the size of tumors on CT scans and/or MRIs to determine growth or shrinkage.

Each of us wants and needs to believe that we will be helped and "cured" by whatever therapy is used. The information you receive from tests results may cause disappointment. However, make certain that you talk to your doctor to ensure that you understand the meaning of terms like "partial response" and "stable disease." These should be viewed as partial successes, not failure. Even if there is no response to a given therapy – a condition known as "stable disease" – this may put you in a holding pattern until a newer treatment or clinical trial is available.

Kidney cancer is too unpredictable, and the therapies are too new, for you to give up fighting because of "stable disease"or "partial response." For this reason, it is important not to let disappointment rob you of your determination or will to live. Simply learn from your experience and go forward with each day.

Seek out a state-of-the-art facility

Patient: Greg
Age: 58

"In June of 2004 I went to see the doctor about what I thought was just a cyst on my scalp. After going through a number of tests, the doctors determined that I had kidney cancer, which had metastasized and was now advanced, including multiple tumors in my lungs. My doctor said it was unlikely I would live to see Christmas.

A local urologist suggested that I visit a clinic out of state that had expertise in kidney cancer, so I went and in August the doctors there took out one of my kidneys, with the thought that it might give me another 19 months. About that time I was doing some Internet research about treatments for kidney cancer and I started reading about the new drugs that were in clinical trials (sorafenib tosylate and sunitinib malate). The closest trial was two states away, but I called them up and asked if I might qualify. Within two weeks I was taking my first pills as a part of the trial. After several cycles of the drug, my lung tumors had decreased by 60 percent, and after six months the doctors couldn't see them anymore. It's been six years since I was diagnosed and I'm still plugging away. I've had some side effects, but they have been manageable.

The hardest thing for me was getting the initial diagnosis of terminal cancer. When they say you have six months to live it is easy to zone out. It floors you. It's hard to find the drive to seek out other options, but somehow I did it.

The real turning point for me was going to a clinic with advanced expertise to have my nephrectomy done. My doctor was extremely caring and involved and I trusted his knowledge. Proactively seeking out a clinical trial was also very important. I felt great afterwards because I feel like my participation in the study may help a lot of other people.

My advice to kidney cancer patients is to educate yourself about the state of the disease because the field is changing so fast, and then find a state-of-the-art care facility. Finding an oncologist with true expertise in kidney cancer is the key."

CHAPTER 5

RADIATION THERAPY

Radiation therapy (RT) is often used when kidney cancer has metastasized to the spine, or other bones, or to the brain. Radiation therapy is used to stop the growth of a tumor, to treat symptoms (e.g., bone pain from a metastasis), and to destroy cancer cells in a bone (e.g., in a fracture, to allow the weakened bone to heal).

How Does Radiation Therapy Work?

DNA is the genetic material inside of all cells, normal and cancerous, which controls the growth and division of cells. Normal cells in the body grow, divide, and die in an orderly fashion. When DNA in a normal cell becomes damaged, it can usually repair itself, but if unable to repair, the individual cell will die. Cancer cells grow and divide despite faulty DNA, continuing to make other abnormal cells. Tumors develop when the abnormal cell growth is out of control. Radiation Therapy disables the DNA of cancer cells, and either destroys the cancer cells or slows their rate of growth.

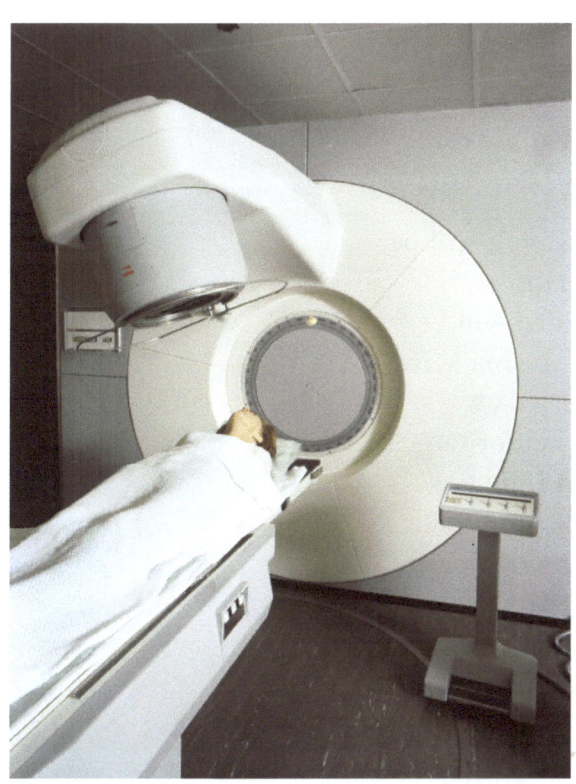

Though not considered a primary form of therapy, various forms of radiation treatment are used to treat certain situations in kidney cancer.

Radiation Therapy is considered a "localized" treatment because it treats a specific area, or "field." The radiation oncologist may recommend RT based on your symptoms, and the number, size, and location of tumors in your body. The total dose of radiation, and the number of treatments (or "fractions"), will be determined by your radiation oncologist. Radiation Therapy may be delivered by different types of machines (e.g., linear accelerators or gamma knife units), but all of them use high energy beams to target tumors as precisely as possible. The beams pass from the machine ("external beam"), and travel through the body to the tumor.

Radiation Therapy for Treatment of Bone and Spine Metastases

Kidney cancer may metastasize to bone (e.g., femur, pelvis, sacrum, humerus), usually causing deep, aching pain in the involved bone, and may also metastasize to the bones of the spine, causing pain and possible neurological symptoms. You should report any new symptoms to your physician immediately. Your physician may order X-rays, a CT scan, or an MRI scan. You may be given a prescription for pain medication or for steroids (e.g., Decadron or Medrol) to help manage symptoms. Your physician may refer you to a radiation oncologist to discuss RT options, or to other specialists who are part of a multidisciplinary team.

Conventional Radiation Therapy (RT)

Conventional RT may also be referred to as "standard" RT, "fractionated" RT, or "external beam" RT. Conventional RT is commonly used to treat bone and spine metastases that are causing pain. It is also used to treat areas of bone that have been weakened by metastases and are at risk of fracture, which may help to keep the bone from breaking. If a fracture does occur, RT may be used to kill cancer cells in the bone and allow the fracture to heal.

When your physician recommends conventional RT, you will be scheduled for a consultation visit, then for a "simulation" appointment. During simulation, the area to be treated will be marked with tattoos, or a mask or other device will be made to hold the area to be treated in the same position every day. Simulation may include a CT scan or X-rays of the tumor target. Radiation Therapy may be given in a single fraction (one large dose), or in a number of smaller doses, usually between three and ten daily treatments or fractions. Your radiation oncologist will need several days to make sure the treatment plan is complete and correct, with the full dose of radiation going to the tumor target, and little or no radiation to other healthy tissues.

During the treatment, you will lie on the treatment table. The radiation therapists line up your tattoos or the marks on the mask/body mold with laser lights that are positioned in the treatment room. You will be placed in the same position for each radiation treatment. The treatment itself lasts only a few minutes. You will not see or feel anything. It is important that you lie very still and breathe normally. As soon as the treatment is over, you may get off the table and leave. You are not radioactive…it is safe for you to be around pregnant women, babies, and small children.

Side Effects of Conventional RT to the Bone and Spine.
Radiation Therapy damages tumor tissue, but may also damage normal healthy tissue, which leads to side effects. Side effects are localized; they occur in the area that was treated (the "radiation field"). Side effects may begin during the course of conventional RT or in the following weeks, and are usually temporary. One of the most common side effects is dry, reddened skin, which may last for 4 to 6 weeks after RT is completed. Your radiation oncology team will provide information about skin care.

Fatigue is a common side effect both during and following RT. Fatigue may be caused by the treatment itself, the combination with other cancer therapies (e.g., targeted therapies or chemotherapy), dietary changes, and by the interruption in daily schedule. Fatigue can last from two to four weeks following completion of RT but sometimes for several months. You should try to pace yourself, get plenty of rest, eat well-balanced, nutritious meals, and get regular moderate exercise to increase your energy.

Sore throat may occur if throat tissues are in the radiation field. Nausea and vomiting or appetite loss may occur if there is esophageal or stomach tissue in the field. Diarrhea may occur if there is bowel in the radiation field, and urinary discomfort if the bladder is in the field. Low blood counts may occur if RT is used to treat metastases in the long bones (pelvis, spine, or femurs). Cough or shortness of breath may occur if there is lung tissue in the radiation field. Your Radiation Oncology team will provide information about symptom management with medications and diet.

Spine Stereotactic Radiosurgery (spine SRS)

A more recently developed alternative to conventional RT for spine metastases is spine stereotactic radiosurgery (spine SRS). Spine SRS uses multiple beams of radiation from many angles. These beams are highly conformed to the tumor target, and deliver a very high dose of radiation, while limiting the dose of radiation to the surrounding healthy tissues. It is very important to avoid normal tissue and the spinal cord in order to prevent injury. Spine SRS is usually delivered in one treatment.

Spine SRS treatment planning is more complex than treatment planning for conventional RT. If your physician recommends spine SRS, you will be scheduled for a high-definition MRI of the area of metastasis in the spine. You will also be scheduled for simulation, and your team will make an immobilization device (a body mold or a mask, depending on the area of the spine to be treated) and obtain a CT scan while you are lying down in the immobilization device. Both the MRI and CT scans are necessary for spine SRS treatment planning, which takes about seven to nine days because of the complexity. When the treatment plan is finalized, you will come in for treatment, and lie on the treatment table in the immobilization device. The accuracy of your position is checked with X-rays, and the treatment is delivered. This takes about an hour, after which you may leave. Your physician will schedule follow up, which may include CT or MRI scans.

Side Effects of Spine SRS. Spine SRS may cause a temporary worsening of your pain, or "pain flare," in the first days following the treatment. The high dose of radiation may cause swelling of the tumor, which puts more pressure on the spinal nerves. This swelling is effectively treated with a short course of steroids (either Decadron or Medrol). You may also continue to take regular pain medications as prescribed. Other side effects of spine SRS depend on the part of the spine that was treated (the radiation field), and may include fatigue, nausea and vomiting, sore throat, diarrhea, or burning with urination. These side effects are generally well managed with medications or diet changes. Keep in touch with your physician or nurse when you are not feeling well.

Radiation Therapy for Treatment of Brain Metastases

Whole Brain Radiation Therapy (WBRT)

Kidney cancer sometimes metastasizes to the brain. Brain metastases may also be treated with radiation therapy, and the decision to use whole brain radiation therapy (WBRT) vs. stereotactic radiosurgery (e.g., Gamma Knife radiosurgery) is based on several criteria, i.e., the size, number, and location of metastatic tumors in the brain. Whole brain radiation therapy delivers relatively small but cumulative doses of radiation to the whole brain, in daily treatment sessions lasting from two to three weeks. These relatively small doses damage tumor DNA, but allow normal brain tissue to repair damage between treatments. If your radiation oncologist recommends WBRT, you will be scheduled for simulation, which includes the making of a mesh mask and a CT scan of your head with the mask in place. Treatment may begin the same day or the following day. During treatment, you will lie on the treatment table with the mask on; treatment usually takes less than 10 minutes per day.

Side Effects of WBRT. Side effects of WBRT include fatigue, which varies from person to person, but may last for several weeks to a few months after treatment is complete. You will likely lose most or all of your scalp hair, which often begins to re-grow within 3 to 6 months after WBRT, although the color, texture, and thickness of new hair may be different. Redness, dryness, and itching to the scalp may occur, and your radiation oncology team will recommend creams, etc., to manage these side effects.

Whole brain radiation therapy may cause some swelling of brain tissues, which may in turn cause other symptoms, most commonly headaches and nausea. Headaches may be managed with over the counter medications such as Tylenol. Nausea may be managed with anti-nausea medications or dietary changes. These side effects sometimes require stronger medications, however, e.g., short term steroids to decrease the swelling in the brain. Hearing changes may occur, sometimes described as "muffled hearing," or "ringing in the ear." This is usually a short term side effect that resolves on its own. You may also develop short term memory problems, and this may be a persistent side effect. Recently, clinical trials have evaluated medications that may be helpful with memory after WBRT.

Stereotactic Radiosurgery for Brain Metastases

Stereotactic radiosurgery may be another treatment option for brain metastases from kidney cancer. This treatment can be delivered using different types of radiation machines, e.g., a linear accelerator, a robotic CyberKnife machine, or a Gamma Knife machine, but the results are very similar whichever treatment machine is used. Gamma Knife Radiosurgery (GKRS) is often a multidisciplinary procedure, with a neurosurgeon and radiation oncologist working together. It is a minimally invasive, outpatient procedure. The Gamma Knife machine uses cobalt as the source of radiation energy, and aims multiple beams of radiation from many different angles at a tumor; these beams intersect at the tumor target and deliver a very high dose of radiation to the tumor. Many cancer centers have the capability to do stereotactic radiosurgery for brain metastases using linear accelerator machines, but the Gamma Knife procedure can only be done at cancer centers with a Gamma Knife (cobalt) machine.

If your oncology team recommends GKRS, when you arrive on treatment day, the neurosurgeon will place a frame on your head, with local anesthesia and IV sedation. The frame is secured with four pins. These pins look much like the tip of a pen, and go through the skin to touch the surface of the skull bones but do not go through the bone. You will have CT and MRI scans done for treatment planning. The frame helps to accurately target the tumor(s) in relationship to the frame. When the treatment plan is finalized and you are ready for treatment delivery, the frame will also keep your head completely still during treatment. When treatment is complete, the head frame is removed, and after a short observation period, you may leave. You may be given a short course of steroids (Decadron or Medrol). You will be scheduled for periodic follow up MRI or CT scans of the brain and to see your physicians.

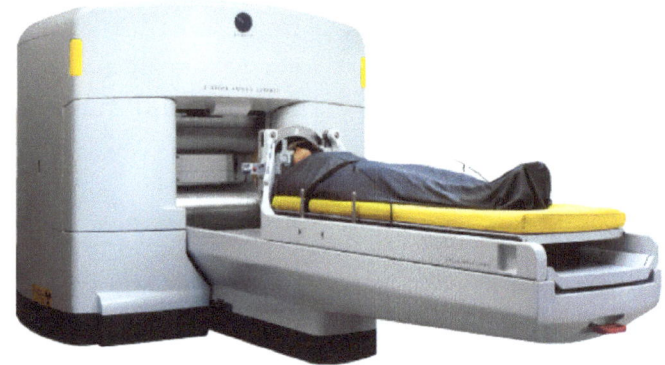
Gamma Knife Unit. (Bing Images)

If your cancer center does not have a Gamma Knife machine, and delivers SRS using a linear accelerator machine or CyberKnife machine, then you will be fitted with a mask for the treatment rather than the head frame.

Side Effects of Stereotactic Radiosurgery for Brain Metastases. Side effects of SRS to the brain may include headaches, nausea, fatigue, and memory changes. The short course of steroids is intended to manage these possible side effects. If you had a head frame for GKRS, you will be instructed in care of the pin sites, and should report any fevers or signs of infection to your physician or nurse. You may lose some hair at the pin sites, but SRS for brain metastases does not cause complete loss of scalp hair. Keep in touch with your physician or nurse if you are not feeling well.

About Steroids

Steroids are anti-inflammatory medications, used to control swelling surrounding a metastasis, and treat the potential symptoms caused by swelling (e.g., headaches, nausea, and pain). Many patients with brain or spine metastases are prescribed steroids. The most commonly prescribed steroid is Decadron (brand name) also known as dexamethasone (generic name). Your physician may start steroids or adjust your steroid dose while you are on radiation treatment, as radiation may cause some additional swelling. For example, if you have headaches, and the headaches worsen, your physician may increase the dose of steroids. Steroids have many side effects, and are intended for short-term use, but it is important to take as directed and to wean the dose gradually.

- Steroids may have an interaction with some targeted therapies. You should discuss steroid use with your oncologist.

- Steroids may cause heartburn. You should take steroids with food. You should also take an acid blocker medication, such as Pepcid (generic name famotidine) to prevent heartburn.

- You may have difficulty sleeping while on steroids. This side effect may wear off if you take your steroid dose(s) no later than mid-afternoon. Your physician or nurse will suggest a schedule for your steroids.

- Steroids may increase your appetite. Try to eat a balanced diet and avoid excessive sweets.

- Steroids may cause your blood sugar to rise, and diabetic patients may need extra insulin. Your endocrinologist will manage this part of your care.

- Steroids may cause external swelling/weight gain around the face and neck, and around the waist and ankles. Most patients lose the extra weight once they are off steroids.

- Steroids may cause mood swings and irritability.

- Steroids may cause a rash to the face or trunk of the body, similar to acne. Wash with a mild hypoallergenic soap, rinse thoroughly, and pat dry.

- At the end of radiation treatment, your physician or nurse will give you a schedule to wean off steroids slowly ("steroid taper"). Your body will need time to adjust to lower and lower doses of steroids. Follow the taper as directed, but call your physician or nurse if you have new or worsening symptoms. Your dose may need to be adjusted, and the taper may need to be slowed down for a while.

About Antioxidants

The use of supplemental antioxidants during cancer treatment is controversial. There are numerous chemical classes of antioxidants, and numerous modes of biologic activity, many of which are not well understood. There is also a wide range in dosages, from the levels found in an adult daily vitamin to high-dose supplements. It is not possible to generalize about how they interact with cancer therapies, or to broadly label all of these supplements as "helpful" or "harmful."

Free radicals react with the DNA in a cell nucleus, and create bonds that may lead to cell damage and death. Antioxidants are compounds that counteract free radicals. They may be produced by the body ("endogenous"), or consumed in antioxidant-rich foods or as supplements. Antioxidants provide benefit by decreasing the formation of free radicals, by acting as scavengers to block free radical damage, and by acting as repair enzymes to reverse damage to cell membranes.

Radiation beams cause damage to tumor cells by "direct hit" to the tumor cell DNA, but also through the process of ionizing the water inside of tumor cells, which causes formation of free radicals and, in turn, further damage to tumor cell DNA.

Some studies have shown that the use of antioxidants during RT or chemotherapy reduces treatment-related side effects, e.g., mouth sores that may occur with RT for cancers of the head and neck. Other studies have shown that high-dose antioxidants can decrease tumor control and shorten survival. There is evidence that antioxidants may protect all cells (normal and tumor cells) from free radical damage during cancer treatment. Still other studies have reported that normal cells are protected better than tumor cells, and that tumor control is not decreased.

Again, the use of supplemental antioxidants during cancer treatment is not well understood, and remains controversial. If you wish to use supplements during your treatment, you should do so only with the approval of your oncology team.

NOTES

Think About Participating in a Clinical Trial

I went to my primary care physician for my yearly physical feeling 'fit as a fiddle.' I had joined a local gym and was exercising with weights and walking two miles a day. During my exam my physician thought that my spleen felt enlarged and asked me to have a scan. Three days later I learned that I had kidney cancer with metastasis. My family and I were in total shock. How could someone who feels so good be so sick? My primary physician advised me to get my things in order. He didn't advise surgery or even chemotherapy because the cancer was so advanced. But after consultation with a surgeon I opted for aggressive treatment. My nephrectomy went smoothly and my surgeon told me I would now be a good candidate for a clinical trial.

Within six weeks from my surgery date I was offered a clinical trial with Interleukin. The treatment was difficult, but it held my cancer stable. I then entered into the Phase III trial with one of the new drugs for kidney cancer that has since been approved by the FDA. My wife and I were nervous because this was to be a "blind" trial. The thought of not knowing if I was getting the drug and the possibility of my cancer progressing was unnerving but the doctor explained that I would be scanned in six weeks and if my cancer was worse I could withdraw from the trial. Anyone who enters a clinical trial has the option of terminating their participation due to progression of their disease or inability to tolerate side effects. I took two pills a day with few side effects and within six weeks my scans showed that my tumors had shrunk. My wife said she had to remind herself that I was a kidney cancer patient in treatment.

Once again the trial drug held my cancer in check for many months until slight growth was detected again. After eighteen months my doctor offered me another trial which I gladly participated in.

I continue to be strongly in favor of clinical trials. I can truthfully say that these clinical trials have given me another chance with a good quality of life. I have told my doctor that I would gladly participate in any clinical trial he recommended. I strongly encourage cancer patients who are eligible to participate in clinical trials. Keep a positive attitude and don't surrender."

CHAPTER 6

CLINICAL TRIALS

*What you should know about participating as a subject
in kidney cancer research*

One of the options for treatment your oncologist may recommend is a clinical trial. Clinical trials are carefully designed research studies that answer specific questions regarding the effectiveness and safety of new drugs, combinations of drugs, surgical techniques, or medical devices. Human volunteers with specific health conditions are studied during the trials to determine the efficacy of the new approaches being tested on them. You may want to consider participating in a clinical trial. Often, trials offer access to promising new treatment options before they are generally available.

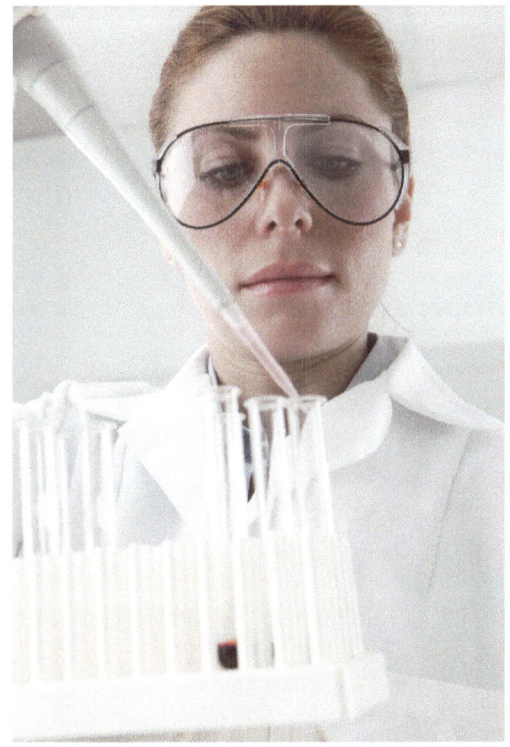

By participating in a clinical trial, you can help advance knowledge to help in the fight against kidney cancer.

Some clinical trials are conducted in "controlled" conditions, meaning that one group of participants receives the therapy being tested and another does not. Later, health information from the two groups is compared to determine if the new therapy had any effect. A key process in such clinical trials is "randomization," in which groups of patients are randomly chosen to receive one treatment or another, thus reducing the chance of bias in the findings.

Clinical trials are conducted by individual institutions (called investigator-initiated trials) or in cooperation with several institutions (called multi-institutional trials) depending on the type of clinical trial and the number of participants that will be enrolled. Clinical trials are organized in cooperation with pharmaceutical companies and with government research organizations such as the National Cancer Institute.

Should You Participate?

Clinical trials have been largely responsible for important advances in the treatment of kidney cancer in recent years. The key to their success is finding suitable human volunteers. By participating, you can obtain access to innovative treatments while helping advance researchers' understanding of kidney cancer. Volunteers in clinical trials play an essential role in the ongoing quest to find a cure for the disease.

Clinical trials are highly regulated and monitored by the Food and Drug Administration. They cannot begin until rigorous intensive review has taken place, in order to ensure the scientific rationale is valid and that there is a fair balance of patient risk and benefit. Still, despite the careful regulation of clinical trials, you should be aware that there are potential drawbacks in addition to the potential benefits of clinical trial participation.

The National Cancer Institute lists the following possible benefits and drawbacks for individuals considering clinical trials.

Potential benefits

- You will receive high-quality health care provided by leading doctors in the field of cancer research.

- You will have access to new drugs and interventions before they are widely available.

- Your health care will be closely monitored, along with any side effects related to the treatment.

- You will play a more active role in your own health care.

- If the approach being studied is found to be helpful, you may be among the first to benefit.

- The trial will provide an opportunity for you to make a valuable contribution to cancer research.

- Depending on the trial, the trial sponsor may pay for some of the medical care or tests required during the trial.

Potential risks

- New drugs and procedures may have side effects or risks unknown to the doctors.

- Side effects and adverse reactions are any undesired actions or effects of the experimental drug or treatment. They may be mild, serious or even life-threatening. They may be worse than those of standard treatment. Experimental treatments are evaluated for bothand long-term side effects.

- New drugs and procedures may be ineffective or may be less effective than current approaches.

- Even if a new approach has benefits, it may not work for you.

- Some health insurance plans prohibit or restrict coverage for clinical trials. Refer to the section titled "Health Insurance" in the chapter "Living With Cancer Day to Day."

- You will have to fit certain requirements of the trial eligibility criteria. Clinical trials have treatment schedules that may require multiple visits to the medical center conducting the trial. This requires a patient to follow a strict calendar that does not allow much flexibility in the treatment schedule.

Types of Clinical Trials

Clinical trials fall into one of several categories:

Phase I Trials

Phase I Trials are the initial studies of a new drug, combination of drugs, or treatment to establish the safest dose. They evaluate the safety of a drug at different doses, and determine if further clinical trials are needed. Most patients participating in Phase I studies have received several types of prior treatment for their cancer. Phase I trials may involve patients with a variety of cancer diagnoses in order to evaluate the safety and determine the appropriate dose and schedule of a drug or treatment in several types of cancer.

Phase II Trials

Phase II Trials are studies which evaluate anti-tumor activity and safety of a drug or treatment in a more defined group of patients at a standard dose and schedule. These studies involve patients with the same type and stage of cancer, and are very specific regarding the type and number of prior treatments that are allowed. For study entry, some Phase II clinical trials do not allow any prior treatment to have been given, and others will require that a specific type of treatment have been given.

Phase III Trials

Phase III Trials compare the effectiveness and safety of two or more treatments in a large number of patients, and may involve up to 1,000 patients. These studies are often international studies, based on the number of patients participating. In Phase III studies, new drugs or treatments are compared with a "standard" treatment in kidney cancer.

"Randomized" clinical trials typically are conducted in Phase III trials, and occasionally in Phase II trials. They compare two or more treatments, and may include a placebo group. Randomized trials are conducted on a large number of patients who are directed into one of the treatment categories using random selection techniques, often by computer. This ensures the validity of the trial results and decreased biases.

A "placebo group" may be included in a Phase II or Phase III trial when there isn't a standard treatment to compare the new drug against. The placebo group receives the same care for cancer and treatment-related symptoms, while allowing the effectiveness of a new therapy to be evaluated. Your oncologist will explain this in more detail if the treatment being recommended involves a placebo group.

Phase IV Trials

The widest-ranging phase of study (usually after the drug/ treatment is commercially available/approved by the FDA) is Phase IV. These trials continue to evaluate the side effects of the drug/treatment, explore new uses of the drug, improved dose schedules, different ways of giving the drug, and the effects of combining the drug with other agents in new, effective regimens.

Eligibility Criteria

The fact that you have kidney cancer doesn't make you automatically eligible for a specific clinical trial. You will have to fit certain requirements of the trial eligibility criteria.

Eligibility criteria for clinical trials are carefully identified to ensure that the group of patients treated has the same type, stage, and extent of cancer. These are referred to as "inclusion" or "exclusion" criteria that must be met in order to be eligible for enrollment into a trial. Specific criteria are listed regarding prior surgery and treatment requirements. Some trials require that patients have had a prior nephrectomy (surgical removal of the kidney tumor) while others do not. Additional criteria are used to ensure that the treatment is appropriate based on organ function. These include laboratory, heart, and lung function, and radiology tests to ensure the safety of subjects.

Selecting a Clinical Trial

It is important for you to understand what a clinical trial is, why it is being done, and how you can gather more information regarding the trial you are interested in. Discuss the trial in detail with your oncologist and nurse and be sure to ask any questions you have regarding treatment and possible participation.

At any time, there may be dozens of clinical trials for kidney cancer. You or your doctor can get a list of current clinical trials by calling 1-800-4-CANCER, or you may look at descriptions of clinical trials at the National Cancer Institute website, www.cancer.gov. The Kidney Cancer Association website, www.kidneycancer.org, offers a free service that will connect you with various other websites offering information about clinical trials. The lists provide a description of each trial, the eligibility criteria, and the name, address, and phone number of the doctor conducting the clinical trial. To find out about a specific trial, have your doctor contact the doctor or nurse conducting the trial – or you may call the study site directly.

Online databases such as MEDLINE contain abstracts of articles published in the journals read by doctors. Your local librarian can help you locate these abstracts, but remember that this information is highly technical and you may want your doctor to review it with you. You should also be aware that because of the time it takes to collect data, prepare a research paper, and have it published, there may not be any published results on the therapy you are considering. In any case, you may want to seek the advice of a kidney cancer specialist before making a final decision to participate in the study. The Kidney Cancer Association can assist you in finding an oncologist who special-izes in kidney cancer. Simply call the Kidney Cancer Association at 1-800-850-9132.

Once you have been given information on treatment options that may include participation in a clinical trial, review the information carefully. Contact the study's doctor (Principal Investigator) and registered nurse (Research Nurse) with any questions you have regarding the treatment options, possible side effects, and frequency of clinic visits. Your doctors and nurses are very interested in helping you be an active member of the team, and can provide you with information that will allow you to make an informed decision regarding your treatment.

Learn to accept your situation and move on

**Patient: Beata
Age: 42**

"Before I was diagnosed with cancer, my life was going great. I had a very nice husband. We had three great kids. We had just bought our dream house. I even had just gotten my dream car. I felt I had it all. I remember I was looking back at my life as I was driving my new car, and I actually started to cry. I just was overcome with emotion and I remember thinking to myself, "God, here I am, a humble person, and I have all this stuff. I never thought in my life I would have all of this." And then, one week later, I was diagnosed with cancer.

I didn't throw my hands in the air and start crying. I tried to adjust and think about it very calmly, even though lots of emotions came through. I never asked "Why me?" If you are going to ask that question you have to also ask "Why not me?" Because realistically, this is something that can happen to any of us.

So my advice to others dealing with kidney cancer is that they shouldn't dwell on questions like, 'Why did this happen to me?' Learn to accept things and move on. Try to think about what's most important in your life – don't get stressed out about things that don't matter. It's a challenge, but at some point it's important to relax and stop worrying. Your emotional or spiritual healing is part of recovering.

CHAPTER 7

HOW TO GET THE MOST FROM YOUR ANTI-CANCER MEDICATION

Believe it or not there are a lot people who do not take their medications as prescribed. The reasons are complex and varied. But the vast majority of those people do not do it deliberately. One study showed that 20% of patients with renal cell cancer did not take their anti-cancer medication properly at least 80% of the time.

How can this happen? There are many reasons, some of which may be familiar.

Cost: As most patients realize, these drugs are expensive. And while there are co-pay assistance programs and other financial assistance programs, not all people are covered all of the time. Individuals may be tempted to skip or reduce doses of their drug to make the supply last longer. (A list of co-pay and financial assistance programs is provided at the end of this chapter.)

Timing of doses can interfere with proper dosing. It may be harder to remember to take a medication twice a day rather than once a day. If a medication needs to be taken on an empty stomach, it may prove difficult to comply. Most individuals take multiple medications, each with its own dosing requirements, such as thyroid medication or supplements, such as magnesium or calcium. Consistently fitting in the anti-cancer medication among all the others may prove difficult.

Side effects: Development of unpleasant side effects or fear of side effects may tempt patients to skip doses. This may be especially true if there is a function or event planned and one does not wish to be plagued by side effects. In addition, the long list of side effects provided by the pharmacy – while meant to be informative – may prompt some patients to question the safety of the medication. In other words, "will this do me more harm than good?"

Work/life responsibilities: These may take priority over one's own needs. That, in combination with convenience or lack thereof, can interfere with proper adherence to the regimen.

Lack of trust in the health care team: If a patent and/or his or her family does not have a trusting and collaborative relationship with the team, studies show the degree of adherence to the prescribed regimen may be in jeopardy.

These are just a few, but not all, of the reasons why patients may not adhere properly to the regimen that has been prescribed. And the major consequence of improper dosing is decreased efficacy. In other words, that drug may not work as well as intended and appear to be ineffective. For this reason your doctor may lose faith in a particular drug and switch therapies, not knowing the real reason is improper dosing.

There are steps patients and their families can take to reduce the risk of improper dosing or non-adherence to the prescribed medication. The first step is for the patient and or family members to become educated about the drug. Research shows that if we are knowledgeable about the medications we take, we are more likely to stick to the proper dosing regimen. To become informed, here are some specific questions that are important to ask:

1. How does the medication work and how can it benefit me?

2. Are there other treatment options for me?

3. What is the proper dosing? For example:

  • How many times a day?

  • With or without food?

  • Can the medication be taken with other medications or supplements?

  • Can the tablet be crushed or the capsule opened?

  • What do I do if I skip a dose?

  • What do I do if I vomit up the medication?

  • What if I take too many doses?

  • Are there other medications or foods I should avoid while taking an anti-cancer medication? (eg: grapefruit, alcoholic beverages, some antibiotics.)

4. What are the side effects and when can I expect to get them?

5. What do I do if I get side effects?

6. How should the medication be stored and are there precautions to take when handling the drug?

7. How often will I have scheduled visits for follow-up?

8. How do I get in touch with my cancer care team during regular hours and on nights and weekends? Phone numbers and/or pager numbers, during clinic hours and after clinic **hours.**

These are important questions to ask prior to starting your anti-cancer medication. Don't be afraid to ask the same questions more than once. It can be hard to absorb all the information in one or two visits. If your clinician does not give you written information that directly addresses your questions, make sure you or a family member write down the information. Some patients bring tape recorders or use the recording device on their smart phones. If you do record the visit, inform your clinician that you are recording the session.

Your cancer care team has a role in helping you manage and properly adhere to your oral anti-cancer medication regimen. To do so, they need to know some things about you and your health.

- At each appointment bring a complete and up-to-date list of all your medications, including non-prescription medications such as vitamins, dietary and herbal supplements. Your medication list should also include a list of any allergies you may have.

- Inform your cancer care team about other health problems you may have, such as high blood pressure, diabetes, or heart disease. Adjusting the dose of your anti-cancer medication may be required.

- Your cancer care team will want to know some additional information about you:

    - What is your living situation?

    - Do you have a spouse or partner?

    - Do you have a good support network?

    - Are you responsible for another person's health and welfare?

- Do you have habits, such as smoking or alcohol use, including beer and wine?

- Do you get regular exercise?

- Provide up-to-date insurance information, including prescription drug coverage. Your cancer care team will help you get financial assistance if needed. Most, if not all, drug companies offer assistance. The team can help you access those programs and others that may be available. Please keep the team informed of any difficulties you may experience in trying to fill your prescription.

- Provide pharmacy information, including a mail order pharmacy if you have one.

Your cancer care team is likely to ask you about all of these things and it is good to be prepared. Also remember to update the team if things change. It is extremely important to inform the team of any new medications prescribed by another provider. Before taking anything new, please check with your cancer care team before filling the prescription. There are many drugs that cannot be taken with anti-cancer medications and your cancer care team can help you find a safer alternative.

There are some practical steps you can take to help you adhere to the proper dosing of your medications in general and your anti-cancer medications in particular.

- Make and keep a list of all the medications you are taking. The list should include the name of the doctor or nurse practitioner who prescribed the medication and their contact information. Keep a copy with you at all times and give a copy to a care giver or family member.

- Use a pill box or pill organizer. This will help you keep track of what you have and have not taken. Most pill cases have compartments for morning and afternoon doses. Make sure a family member or care giver knows your medication schedule too. That is why it is helpful if that person has an up-to-date list.

- Create a pill diary or calendar that includes the exact dates and times of the doses and record when you have taken them.

- Establish a reminder system. There are medication reminder apps for smart phones and most are free. Many of these apps allow you to set reminders for multiple medications, help keep track of refills and provide information on drug interactions. (Included at the end of this chapter is a partial list of apps.) Setting an alarm can be helpful if you do not have a smart phone. Taking your medication at the same time every day can serve as a reminder, especially if you take it in conjunction with another daily routine, such as brushing your teeth.

- Plan ahead for refills. Keep an eye on how many pills you have left and the number of refills allowed on the prescription. Ideally, refills should be requested about 7 to 10 days before the prescription will run out. Many mail-order pharmacies keep track of this for you. However, you shouldn't rely solely on the pharmacy's system and should be aware of when you are going to run out of medication and will need a refill.

- Report and manage side effects. As mentioned previously, you may be tempted to skip or reduce the dosage if bothered by side effects. This may prevent you from getting the full benefit of the anti-cancer medication. Prompt reporting of side effects and following through on treatment recommendations can reduce the risk of side effects interfering with your quality of life.

- Keep follow-up appointments. These appointments are important for monitoring your response to treatment.

- Communication is key. Many patients may be reluctant to report side effects or new health problems for fear of being taken off the anti-cancer medication. Quite often, holding or reducing doses is recommended. This is a normal part of managing anti-cancer medications. Your cancer care team will work with you to maintain the right cancer care for you. Don't be afraid to ask questions!

Adherence to your prescribed anti-cancer drug regimen is essential for getting the full benefit from the treatment. Knowledge is power: knowing about the drug, what it can do and cannot do, knowing how to properly dose the medication and knowing how to actively manage the side effects are key. Establishing a reminder system, involving your family or caregiver and keeping an open and honest line of communication with your cancer care team will all serve you well for optimizing your cancer care.

Patient Resources

Smartphone App Medication Reminders

This is just a small sampling of the apps available. Visit your App store for complete information and to find the one that works best for you:

- *Pill Reminder - All in One*: Free, iOS
- *Drugs.com Medication Guide*: Free, iOS, Android
- *MediReminder*: $3, Blackberry and Android
- *Dosecast - Medication Reminder:* Free, iOS and Android
- *MediSafe Meds and Pill Reminder:* Free, iOS and Android
- *Pillboxie:* $0.99, iOS and Android

Associations and Professional Groups

Kidney Cancer Association: www.KidneyCancer.org

American Cancer Society: 800-227-2345 www.cancer.org

National Coalition for Cancer Survivorship: 877-622-7937
     www.canceradvocacy.org

Cancer.net/American Society of Clinical Oncology
     www.cancer.net

Patient Assistance Programs

Pharmaceutical Industry

Pfizer Rx Pathways: 866-706-2400 pfizerrxpathways.com
     (Sutent, Inlyta)

REACH program: 866-6392827 www.nexavar-us.com
     (Nexavar)

Patient Assistance Now Oncology: 866-884-5906
     www.oncologyaccessnow.com
     (Afinitor)

GSK for you: 866-518-4357 www.gskforyou.com
     (Votrient)

Independent Charities

CancerCare: 866-552-6729 www.cancercarecopay.org

Chronic Disease Fund: 877-968-7233 www.cdfund.org

Patient Access Network Foundation: 866-316-7263
www.panfoundation.org

Patient Advocate Foundation: 866-512-3861 www.copays.org

Healthwell Foundation: 800-675-8416
www.healthwellfoundation.org

Advocate for yourself and explore all the options

Patient: Rick
Age: 55

"What I have learned is that with kidney cancer, it's important to become your own advocate. You have many choices after diagnosis, and you should do everything you can to educate yourself and get the care that is best suited for your case. Knowledge is power.

I was told after my initial radical nephrectomy that the surgeon "had gotten it all." I returned to the life of a 50-year-old male, busy with career and family. It was 18 months later that the tumors were found in my lungs and I was now living with Stage IV, metastatic renal cell cancer. My oncologist's plan of action after the second diagnosis seemed tentative, but I hesitated to change doctors or seek out another opinion because I didn't want to be disloyal.

Through the action and influence of my wife, we consulted an oncologist at a cancer center in our state, along with two leading experts in the nation. The oncologist at the cancer center recommended IL2 and the two experts concurred. That gave me confidence that we were doing the right thing. I went through the high-dose IL2 therapy and I feel it has been influential in bringing me up to my fifth year of survival.

I've learned that cancer care is not consistent and it is not standardized. I was in a kind of emotional fog when I was diagnosed and at the first wasn't really motivated to seek out information and alternatives. Thanks to my wife I was able to shake off the lethargy and take action. I'm convinced that the reason I am here today is through empowerment and a proactive search to find the right oncologist, the right hospital and the right therapy."

CHAPTER 8

PATIENT EMPOWERMENT

*Patients and families have rights, responsibilities,
and many options as they face kidney cancer. Here are important
empowering steps you should take following your diagnosis.*

One way you can increase your odds of survival after a diagnosis of kidney cancer is by becoming a strong self-advocate in all phases of your care.

Remember that you and your family have options and rights – as well as responsibilities – at every step of the way as you deal with your cancer. By exercising your options, rights, and responsibilities, you will become empowered and be able to make sound decisions. And your peace of mind will increase.

Here are the basic steps to empowerment and increasing your odds of surviving.

Self Advocacy

Don't Rush

Do not rush into surgery or treatment without getting some basic facts about your specific type of cancer. Your doctor and your emotions may be telling you to act quickly. But your tumor has been part of you for months, perhaps even years. Not all types of cancer are fast growing. Take your time to get a few basic facts so you can make informed decisions. First steps might impact your disease course or future treatment options. Time is important, but it is more important to get the right care than to save a few days or a week.

Get the Facts

It's important to become informed about your diagnosis and options as early as possible. A good first step is to go to libraries or search the Internet for disease information. Visit a hospital patient library or a medical school library. Read medical journals if you have a technical background. Or get your local public library to do a computerized literature search for information on your disease. Many libraries will search for you free of charge. You can see which doctors are doing the most research, and you can consider getting a second opinion regarding treatment options. Be sure to review the patient resources section included in this book.

The Internet is a great source of information, but remember that some of what you may find could be inaccurate. You may find information that is taken out of context or may not apply to your situation. This can lead to both false hope and unfounded fear. As you search, rely on sites that are known for providing accurate, credible information. Every patient is an individual and the course of your disease will not be exactly like that of other patients. Be wary of making comparisons between yourself and others with the same diagnosis while searching online. Checking facts and validating understanding is important.

Contact Your Patient Organization

The Kidney Cancer Association (KCA) serves kidney cancer patients and offers information that can be helpful to you. In addition to this book, KCA distributes a free monthly email newsletter, *Kidney Cancer News*. A quarterly publication, *Kidney Cancer Journal*, is distributed to doctors' offices and it may be accessed at the KCA website, www.kidneycancer.org.

You may also contact the American Cancer Society at 1-800-ACS-2345. The U.S. Centers for Disease Control & Prevention website (www.cdc.gov) publishes a list of cancer information links.

Finally, look for a local cancer patient support group or patient advocacy meeting in your community and attend. You can learn more about finding a kidney cancer support group or meetings by calling the Kidney Cancer Association at 1-800-850-9132 or by visiting the website at www.kidneycancer.org.

Get a Second Opinion

Finding a doctor who specializes in your type of cancer is a good idea. Your doctor may be an excellent physician, but some types of cancer are very rare so your doctor may not see enough cases to be good at treating your disease. In medicine, practice makes perfect.

Start by asking your doctor for a referral for a second opinion. Don't hesitate to take this step – doctors aren't upset if you get a second opinion, and this is your right and responsibility.

You can find an expert doctor by asking the Cancer Information Service or the Kidney Cancer Association for the names and phone numbers of experts in your area. Call one or two expert doctors and make appointments to see them. Sometimes, these "super doctors" are very busy and you may need a referral from a cancer patient organization. Ask for this help.

Your Responsibilities

Keep Good Records

Get in the habit of collecting reports and records at the time of visits to doctors or other health professionals, and keep everything organized. You will want to keep pathology reports from all surgeries and/or biopsies, reports from scans and CDs of images and other tests, and records of any treatments given. A binder with separation tabs is an ideal way to organize your health information and medical or surgical reports.

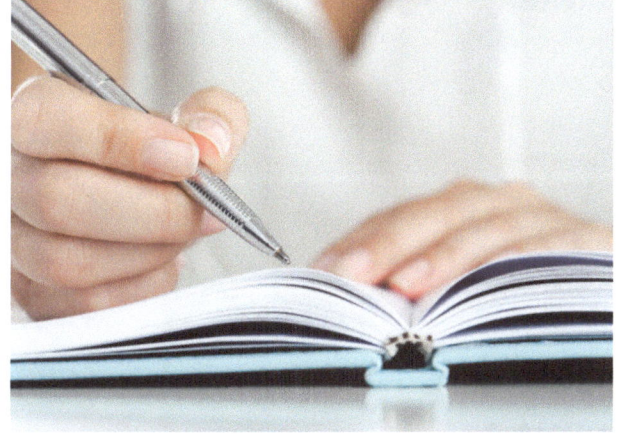

One of the most important things you can do as a patient is ensure that you keep your medical records well organized and up to date. A personal medical journal may be helpful.

Bring these records to any new appointment, especially one in which you are receiving a second opinion. Take films or a CD with your most recent scans to the visit (don't leave them there unless the doctor asks you to.) Keep an updated, legible list of all your medications, and provide the doctor with a copy. Be sure to include any "over the counter" medications and complementary therapies.

You are entitled to copies of your medical, surgical, and pathology records. Do not be surprised if the doctor asks you to sign a receipt for your x-rays or charges you for copying documents. A receipt is simply a written record that you were given the materials you requested. Don't hesitate to ask for your records. If you have any trouble obtaining them, contact the hospital ombudsman.

Hire an Expert

Get the most qualified doctor to treat you. Do not confuse "bedside manner" with true expertise. You want to be given the most appropriate treatment, not be charmed.

You are more likely to find an expert doctor at a comprehensive cancer center associated with a university medical center, particularly for a rare type of cancer. However, there are many excellent doctors in community hospitals. Do not hesitate to be treated by them if they have experience with your type of disease. Simply ask your doctor how many patients with your type of cancer he or she has treated in the past 12 months. Then compare this number with the other doctors you are researching.

Some medical centers are famous. However, when it comes to rare cancers, a less well-known cancer center may offer more advanced care and have more doctors who are experts in your type of cancer.

Be sure to ask for statistics measuring surgical success, morbidity, and rates of complications associated with treatments.

Communicate Professionally With Your Doctor

Establishing good communications with your doctor is essential to a good outcome, and good communication is a **shared** responsibility. To start, fax all records you have prior to your visit, and take your records with you. You may also want to send a letter or fax telling your doctor about any changes in your medical condition since your last visit. Include new symptoms such as pains, bleeding, any new illnesses such as colds, and any crises in your life such as getting fired. Ask your doctor for a "point person" in the office for your questions, and determine the preferred method – e-mail, fax, phone, etc.

If you use a phone to communicate with your doctor or nurse and deliver a message, be proactive and call back if you have not received a response in a reasonable amount of time. Phone messages sometimes do not go through or the voice mail may not be clear and your message may not be heard. Do not assume that your message is being ignored. Call back to double check that your message got through. If you leave a message on a voice mail, include as much identifying information as you can. Large clinics have many patients, some with similar names. The more information you give in your message, the faster your nurse or doctor will be able to identify you and respond to your questions or concerns.

It's always a good idea to have questions written down before your visit. Be honest and clear with your questions, and be straightforward in all of your communications with your doctor. You have the right to expect honest, clear responses. If possible, take an advocate with you to help with note taking and for support.

By taking these steps, you will be better prepared to meet your doctor. Your doctor should be able to answer your questions, and should be receptive to your active participation in the determination of the best treatment plan for you. This business-like approach will make your doctor respect you. It will also set the tone for your patient-doctor relationship. If your doctor will not answer your questions, find another doctor. You are entitled to clear communications.

Be a Skeptic

Your surgeon will not be able to guarantee that "I got it all." If you are treated surgically, you should be skeptical of such a claim. What the surgeon really means is that he or she removed all of the tumor that could be seen. If your surgeon did not see it, it wasn't removed.

Some tumors have many blood vessels. Tiny bits of tumor or even a few cancer cells can drift off in the bloodstream and settle elsewhere in your body. Years after your primary tumor is removed, these cells can form new tumors that may need to be treated. You will need regular medical check-ups. If a new tumor starts up, you want to catch it early and treat it promptly. **Never let your guard down.** Make sure you get regular follow-up care.

Be Accountable for Your Follow-up

Don't assume that someone at your doctor's office is responsible for your follow-up. You should take responsibility for getting a follow-up visit scheduled and for keeping the appointment.

Get regular follow-up testing, which might include CT scans, bone scans, and blood tests. Get the results of these tests in writing, and ask for a referral or see an expert for abnormal findings. If you are uncomfortable with abnormal findings that your doctor is not treating, ask for a second opinion.

Appeal and Hang Tough

Today's health care insurance system can be complicated. Again, remember that you have rights and options, but also responsibilities. An important first step is finding a financial representative or billing counselor at the institution that will be submitting bills related to your care (hospital, medical group, etc.). Communicate clearly and professionally with this person, who could end up being your best ally. Work with all billing and reimbursement parties to set up ongoing payment plans that are reasonable and ensure your credit will be protected.

Appeal any insurance claim that is rejected. Your ability to get state-of-the-art care can be influenced by your insurance coverage. If a claim is rejected, resubmit it. Another claims reviewer at your insurance company may evaluate your claim differently and authorize payment. Be persistent.

Every insurance company has a claims appeal process. If your claim continues to be rejected, you can contact your state insurance commission and patient organization for assistance. Sometimes, a call to an insurance company medical director from a patient organization can help get your claim paid.

Be reasonable. Do not expect your insurance company to pay duplicate claims, fraudulent claims, claims which are not covered by your policy, or claims for unproven treatments. Since you are a policyholder, your insurance company pays claims with your money. You want your insurance company to have a fair review process but not an unreasonable one.

Don't Play Doctor

Don't take vitamins, herbal preparations or other medications without talking to your doctor. Many patients want to help themselves. Vitamin supplements and good nutrition may have a role to play in cancer care. However, large doses of some supplements can interfere with some drugs or radiation therapy. Do not medicate yourself, even if you are a doctor. Excellent nutrition information is available from the American Institute for Cancer Research.

Do not throw away money on treatments which have no medical justification. Some alternative therapies are based on sound theories. However, without scientific knowledge and investigating details, you will not be able to tell which ones have some validity and which are exploiting vulnerable patients.

If your cancer does not respond to the first treatments you try, discuss this with your doctor and move on to the next one. There are many valid therapies for every type of cancer. New ones are being developed constantly.

Join and Be Active

Join a cancer patient organization that specializes in your type of cancer. Many organizations provide emotional support for cancer patients. But don't settle for emotional support alone. You want to beat cancer, not just feel good emotionally. If you read popular books on cancer, remember the real message about emotional support: "Good mental health is necessary for good physical health." But do not expect tumors to just disappear because you have engaged in guided imagery, meditation, relaxation, or some other self-help technique.

The best organizations have ongoing information programs for patients. For example, the Kidney Cancer Association publishes a monthly e-newsletter and holds conferences for patients and doctors.

Science is making tremendous progress in many types of cancer. Stay informed. Get involved. Meet other informed patients. Meet the doctors and scientists who are true experts in your type of cancer. If you have a recurrence, you will know what your treatment options are and who can give you the best care. Be an activist; support the patient organization so it can support you. Act in your own self-interest.

Seek and Ask

Continually seek information. If a doctor tells you a tumor is inoperable, get a second opinion. Call the Cancer Information Service to get a list of clinical trials for your type of cancer. When you get the list, review it with your doctor. Ask why this proposed trial is best for you. Talk with other patients who have had any proposed therapy so you know what to expect. If there are side effects, remember not all patients get every side effect. Ask your doctor what he or she can do to control side effects.

Summary

Patient empowerment leads to a better understanding of your disease, a stronger sense of control over your cancer, and the best approach to treating your kidney cancer. There are many resources available to help you and your family adjust to the diagnosis. Don't be afraid to ask about them.

You are part of the team in deciding on your treatment plan. You have rights and responsibilities as a patient. You need to work with your doctor and the rest of your health care team to maximize your care and make use of resources available to you.

Families can make all the difference

(Jason's father was diagnosed with kidney cancer)

"Since his diagnosis, my dad had his kidney removed. He's in a clinical trial now, and doing well.

A cancer diagnosis is a challenge for a family. My father needed help in understanding medical terms and instructions so someone had to be there with him at all of the appointments. And we had to organize all of the medical records for him. I ended up being the person who did most of the coordinating, as my other brothers couldn't get away as much.

My advice for any family members helping someone with kidney cancer is: Get super-organized. We bought a large artist's portfolio with zipper sides and carrying handles and kept all of my dad's X-rays and medical records in it. We just carried it with us to every appointment. And I kept very detailed records in a notebook of every conversation. I wrote down everybody's names, the dates and times and what they said in the meetings. Things can move pretty fast in a medical meeting and it's easy to forget details.

Beyond the practical side, I think it's also very important for families to talk to each other a lot when dealing with cancer. You have to accept the fact that someone in the family is sick and talk about your feelings openly. Try to stay close to each other and when you have a problem, talk about it. Sometimes men don't want to show their feelings as much, but you have to have a release.

The biggest challenge is not knowing whether the cancer will recur, and that means a sense of hope becomes very important. You have to move on after the diagnosis and concentrate on the positive things. If you dwell on the negative you will never get through it. For me, that means being more spiritually involved. Others might find hope another way, but you have to find it somewhere."

CHAPTER 9

LIVING WITH CANCER DAY TO DAY

The impact of kidney cancer on your life is complex. Here are suggestions on what to expect – from employment matters and health insurance to diet, lifestyle, and family relationships.

As you learn more about kidney cancer, and perhaps meet other kidney cancer patients, you will see that it is possible to live a full and satisfying life after your diagnosis. But your life will obviously be impacted, both during your initial treatments and during your recovery phase.

Supportive Care

As you adjust to your diagnosis, you may deal with a number of physical, emotional, and practical issues that could pose challenges. It is important to remember that dealing with these issues is a central part of your overall care – and resources are available to help. This component of your overall health plan is called Supportive Care, and it encompasses all forms of care aimed at supporting your quality of life.

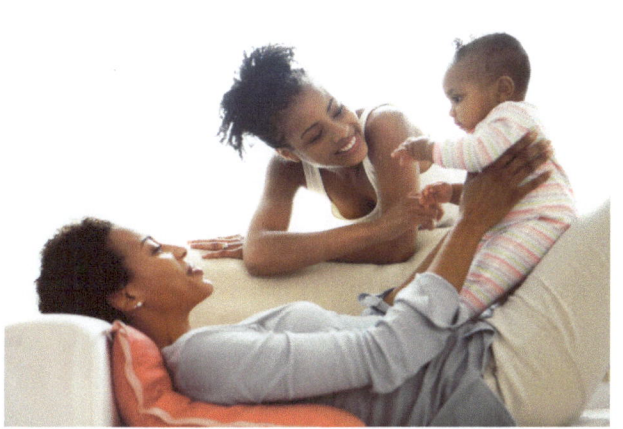

Kidney cancer can have a major impact on your home life. Building an atmosphere of open communication and support helps the patient progress in recovery.

Among the important psychosocial support elements of Supportive Care are management of nausea, pain, fatigue, nutrition, exercise and physical therapy, family life, and practical matters such as health insurance. As you begin to create a Supportive Care plan, be sure to have frank discussions with your doctor and health care team at any time you feel anxious or uncertain about what you should do. An expert oncology team should be able to address any of these issues, providing care or making a referral for help. (Information about end-of-life issues, palliative care, and hospice are included in the chapter "Emotional Well-Being.") As you learn more about dealing with your disease, remember that each type of cancer has unique properties and symptoms. Be aware that advice and support that may be helpful for one type of cancer patient may not apply to someone with kidney cancer.

Nausea, Pain, and Fatigue

Cancer patients often have to deal with nausea, pain, and fatigue – which have a multitude of causes. Some are related directly to the cancer itself, others to the treatment that kidney cancer patients receive. Not everyone experiences these symptoms, but if you do, treatment is available.

Nausea. Nausea may have a number of causes, including systemic treatment (immunotherapy, chemotherapy, targeted therapy) or radiation treatments, tumor growth, or anxiety about your disease. A variety of strategies aimed at reducing nausea yourself may be attempted, ranging from eating smaller meals to drinking smaller amounts of fluids more frequently, and trying such things such as relaxation exercises and meditation. If these techniques are not effective, your doctor might prescribe anti-nausea medicine. Also known as anti-emetics, anti-nausea medicines are usually taken orally and can significantly reduce symptoms of nausea. Many are available, and various kinds or combinations can be tried until a successful combination is found.

Pain. If you experience pain, it may be related to your kidney cancer itself or to some of the treatments you might receive. You should always communicate clearly and honestly with your health care team about any pain you might be experiencing. Describe the quality of your pain – that is, where does it fall on a scale of 0 to 10 (0 being "no pain" and 10 being "the worst imaginable pain")? Where is the location of the pain? Is it constant or does it only happen occasionally? Does anything make your pain increase or lessen (i.e. change in body position to lying, sitting, standing; application of heat or cold to the painful area)?

Working with your doctor and health care team, you may want to establish goals for treating your pain. Consider what activities you need to be able to do to improve the quality of your life (helping your children with homework after school, for example). Many pain medications are available to control pain – both prescription and over-the-counter. Note: Fear of addiction to pain medication can lead to unnecessary distress, pain, and not being able to do things that are important to you. This fear is not valid, as there are very few "addiction issues" in cancer patients. It is very important to discuss this and other concerns you have about pain medication with your doctor and nurse.

Some patients with cancer may think that being on pain medications means that they are near the end of their life. This is not necessarily true. If this is a worry or concern, please let your doctor know – he or she can explain the use of pain medication in your recovery plan. Pain medications can be supplemented or in some cases replaced by non-medical interventions such as meditation and relaxation therapies.

Fatigue. Fatigue is one of the most distressing side effects of cancer, and can significantly impact your life. Fatigue may be caused by many factors, including depression, insomnia, anemia (below-normal levels of red blood cells), the effects of cancer treatment, and changes in your body's metabolism caused by your cancer. Treatment-related fatigue is quite common.

To combat fatigue, patients are advised to pace their activities and prioritize where they want to expend their energy. Organizing your home and work environment in a way that helps accommodate your lower energy levels can help, and you should try to limit your physical demands before, during, and after treatment for kidney cancer. Treatment for anemia can help, as can exercise regimens, nutrition, and stress management techniques. Drug therapy for fatigue is occasionally used. Be sure to discuss your level of fatigue with your health care team and discuss possible solutions.

Constipation. It is not unusual for cancer patients to become constipated. Contributing factors are pain medications, cancer treatment, lack of exercise, and poor nutrition. In many cases, nutritional adjustments and increased intake of water can be very helpful. Other approaches are also available – again, discussion with your health care team is an important first step.

Depression. It is not unusual for cancer patients to become depressed. Current low-dose antidepressants are safe, well tolerated and effective as treatment. Use of antidepressants should not be considered a sign of weakness – they are an important part of an overall treatment plan for some patients.

The Role of Diet and Nutrition

After a diagnosis of cancer, it is natural to think about diet and nutrition. Family, friends and co-workers will want to offer advice, which may include eating exotic foods or supplements. You may read about herbs or vitamins which claim to help fight cancer. There may also be confusing information on the Internet. The best rule of thumb is to discuss your diet, goals and any new food ideas first with your kidney cancer doctors or nutritionist. Most hospitals have nutrition experts who can give you practical advice.

The precise relationship between diet and kidney cancer is unknown. However, diet has been estimated to be a causal factor in about 35% of all cancers. Some people think a high-protein diet might be a risk factor. Obesity also may play a role in kidney cancer, as it does in other cancers.

The American Institute for Cancer Research advises to mostly eat plant foods, limit red meat and avoid processed meat (examples are ham, bacon, hot dogs and beef jerky). Intake of processed meats has been linked to cancer because of the carcinogens that can form during the preserving process. Other recommendations include avoiding salty foods, such as canned soups, pizza, and frozen meals, and limiting daily salt intake to less than 2400 milligrams (1 teaspoon).

There is limited scientific evidence showing that certain foods or a change in diet or supplements will slow the growth of kidney cancer that is already present. However, a healthy diet and exercise will help promote strength, energy, a healthy immune system, improved mood and regeneration of normal tissues. Eating a well balanced diet is especially important if you are undergoing cancer therapy.

Some foods, such as garlic, have shown protective properties against stomach cancer. Studies have shown that certain foods contain power-packed nutrients for overall health and preventing some types of cancers. Some of these outstanding foods include dark leafy green vegetables, soybeans, grapes, green tea, cruciferous vegetables such as broccoli, and flaxseed.

Some patients become vegetarians or adopt a macrobiotic diet. Such a diet may be beneficial as long as it is properly balanced and meets your nutritional needs. Adhering to a specific diet regimen may make you feel like you have more "control" over your disease. But, again, there is little evidence that a change in diet will affect how your kidney cancer grows and some diets can actually be harmful or distracting at a time when you need energy to fight your cancer. Do not start eating new or strange fruits or foods from other countries before you ask your doctor, because they may contain ingredients which decrease the effect of your cancer medicine or other medicines.

Vitamins and Herbal Supplements

Many cancer patients medicate themselves with nutritional supplements. For example, some patients take megadoses of vitamins in the belief that they will prevent recurrence or even cure their cancer. There is little research evidence that such self-medication can directly influence recurrence or cure.

Patients should exercise extreme caution in using vitamins and herbal supplements. Studies show that taking megadoses of some vitamins or supplements, such as vitamin A or vitamin E, can be damaging to health.

Supplements that contain vitamin A may interact with some drugs to produce unwanted side effects and toxicity. They can also cause liver toxicity or damage when taken in combination

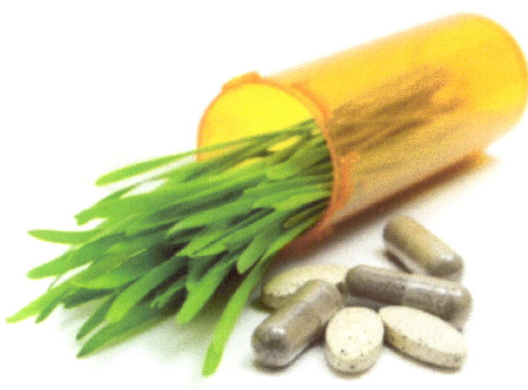

with other retinoids (substances related to vitamin A). Another example of a supplement that can interfere with medicine is St. John's Wort.

Patients should also recognize that dietary supplements sold in health food stores are not regulated by the U.S. Food and Drug Administration (FDA). All processed food products, all prescription drugs, and all over-the-counter drugs sold in the U.S. are regulated by the FDA. Manufacturing plants for these products are also inspected by the FDA.

While there are many good manufacturers of dietary supplements, you cannot be certain of the quality of supplements. For example, all prescription drugs are date coded and may not be sold after a certain period of time to ensure effectiveness and safety. Dietary supplements are not necessarily date coded, and it is difficult to know if a product on the shelf of a health food store is fresh. Companies that make these products are not inspected by the FDA.

Do not start taking megadoses of vitamins, new vitamins, or other nutritional supplements without first talking with your doctor. Some patients do not want their doctor to know about their use of these products because they fear that he or she won't approve. In reality, every experienced doctor has worked with patients who have taken supplements. Your doctor won't be surprised if you express an interest in nutritional supplements.

While your doctor may not be a nutritional expert, a frank discussion may prevent you from making a serious mistake or help you avoid a dangerous drug interaction. If you want to pursue nutritional strategies, seek out a physician who is an expert at nutrition research.

A healthy, well-balanced diet that includes fruits, vegetables, legumes (beans), fiber, whole grains (such as oatmeal, brown rice, whole wheat bread, and whole grain cereals) and lean protein (such as fish and chicken without fat) should provide the vitamins and minerals needed by most people. Taking extra vitamins or herbal supplements will usually not be needed if you are eating healthy foods.

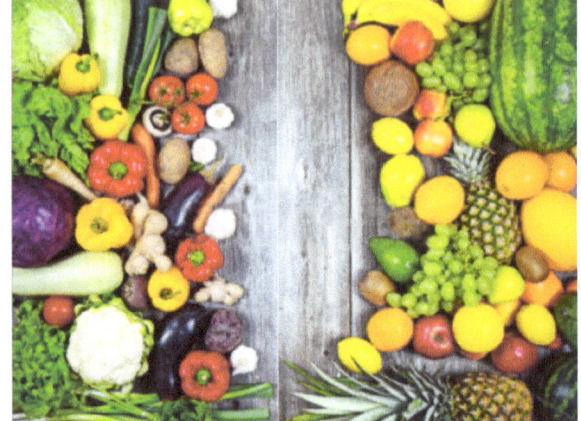

Patients who have had a nephrectomy usually have one functioning kidney and half their normal renal capacity. The kidney must adjust and filter the blood and substances within the bloodstream. Always inform your doctor that you have only one kidney, as this can affect any future medication prescription that may be ordered for you.

To help your other kidney process blood and its components after a nephrectomy, you should drink plenty of water. You can also help yourself by avoiding drinks with high sugar content such as sweet tea and soft drinks. Your doctor will check your bloodwork to make sure your kidney is working well.

If you are overweight, be sure to discuss your weight with your oncologist before starting a weight-loss plan. Your doctor may be able to give you guidance for a plan to lose weight that does not negatively affect you or your treatment plan.

Patients often wonder if they can drink alcoholic beverages after having a kidney removed for kidney cancer. The answer is "yes." A social drink now and then, a beer at a sporting event, or wine with a special dinner probably won't hurt you. Discuss this with your doctor, as it may not be recommended at specific times during treatment. After cancer has disrupted your life, such simple pleasures become more meaningful. There is even some medical research evidence that suggests that a glass of wine on a regular basis may have health benefits. You may also find the new non-alcoholic beers to your liking. Beverages brewed from whole grains can have nutritional value.

Some common questions received by patients include:

Q: **My cousin told me about a fruit from Mexico that kills cancer. Can I eat this?**

A: Since we do not know the ingredients, it is best to avoid an exotic fruit like this and stick to the ones we know are good, such as strawberries and blueberries. The fruit from Mexico could contain chemicals which we do not know about and could interfere with your other medications or harm your liver.

Q: **How much protein should I eat each day since I only have one kidney?**

A: The average person gets 15% protein from their daily calories. As long as your creatinine is within the normal range, your kidney can break down the average amount of protein in your daily diet.

Q: **Should I use supplement drinks or shakes?**

A: Yes, they are allowed as long as your kidney function (creatinine) is within the normal range. It is not recommended to use protein drinks or shakes as a routine diet supplement. Some of the powders contain more protein than your body needs. Consult your nutritionist, who can review different protein supplements or drinks with you.

Q: **There is an herbal tea I want to try, will this be OK?**

A: Check with your doctor first.

Q: **Do I need to follow a special diet to preserve my functioning kidney?**

A: There is no special diet recommendation, except for some people who have other health concerns, such as diabetes or high blood pressure. For everyone, the suggested dietary lifestyle is to maintain a healthy weight, avoid excess salt and avoid processed or refined foods (doughnuts, boxed dinners) and high sodium convenience foods (canned goods or frozen dinners). Daily nutrition should include a high intake of whole foods (fruits, vegetables, nuts/seeds, legumes and lean animal protein).

Additional information about the role of diet and nutrition in cancer, including downloadable brochures and pamphlets, can be found on the American Institute for Cancer Research website (www.aicr.org). You can also find materials at the National Cancer Institute website (www.cancer.gov), and a variety of other websites. See the Resources section at the end of this book.

Complementary and Alternative Medicine (CAM)

Some patients believe that "conventional" medicine will not cure their cancer. They think that "toxic" treatments will damage their immune system. These patients do not appreciate how immunotherapy works or how advanced scientific cancer care has become.

You may have heard about shark cartilage as a cancer treatment. There is no research evidence that eating shark cartilage works. The same holds true for bovine cartilage, another alternative treatment.

Some patients try essiac tea, a brew made from tree bark and herbs. Essiac contains some interesting chemicals, but there is no research evidence that it can cure cancer or prevent recurrence.

Herbs have been used in medicine for centuries. In fact, most pharmaceutical preparations were originally made from plants until the 1950s, when organic chemistry was developed, leading to the synthesis and manufacture of naturally occurring chemicals. Taxol, a drug used to treat ovarian cancer, was originally made from the bark of the Pacific Yew tree until it could be synthesized.

Many herbs cannot be simply ingested. They must be prepared to release their active ingredients and make them biologically available in the body. In addition, some herbs can interact with other medications. Without adequate knowledge, you can injure yourself.

Some patients try going to cancer clinics in Mexico, the Bahamas, or Europe. There is no evidence that treatments available in these clinics offer any therapeutic advantage over what is available at cancer centers in the United States. Moreover, your insurance is not likely to reimburse you for care at these clinics. Some of them may also engage in unethical and dangerous medical practices.

For example, coffee enemas to "de-toxify" patients have caused colon ruptures, resulting in serious infections and death. Another remedy contained rattlesnake meat which was found to be contaminated by rare bacteria related to tuberculosis. Several patients died as a result of that remedy.

More information about Complementary and Alternative Medicine is available from the website of the National Center for Complementary and Alternative Medicine (www.nccam.nih.gov). See the Resources section at the end of this book for other related information.

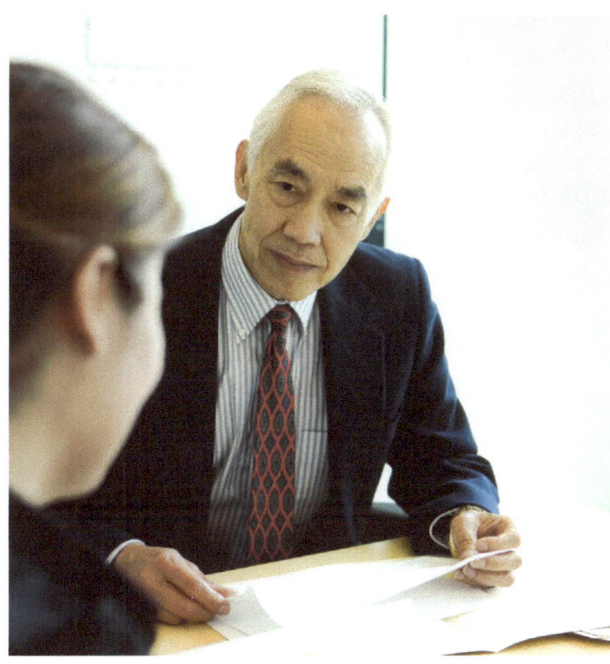

Issues of health insurance and employment can be difficult to deal with while your mind is occupied with your cancer. It's important to become familiar with the details of your insurance and employer policies.

Smoking

If you smoke, stop and never smoke again. Smoking is one of the risk factors for kidney cancer. Get professional help by asking your doctor to recommend a smoking cessation program. If you are worried about gaining weight, stop smoking anyway and deal with any possible weight gain through diet and exercise. Encourage people around you, especially young people, to stop smoking cigarettes or avoid starting.

Exercise

Exercise is good for you. After surgery, modest exercise can help you regain your muscle tone and help rebuild the muscles that were cut. Exercise can complement dieting, making it easier to lose weight.

Try to get at least one half hour of exercise every other day. Vigorous walking, jogging, swimming, or other aerobic exercise promotes good cardiovascular health and may help reduce high blood pressure. Walking is an excellent form of exercise if done regularly.

Exercise is also a good way to reduce and manage stress. Regular exercise is also thought to slow down the aging process. Unfortunately, in modern society where many people work in sedentary jobs, we often don't get enough exercise. Try to make time for regular daily exercise and to make it a part of your lifestyle.

You can start out with slow and easy exercise, gradually increasing the amount until you achieve your goals. Always consult with your doctor before embarking on an exercise program so changes in levels of fatigue can be accurately monitored and fragile bones and/or muscles will not be stressed.

Family Life

Kidney cancer will probably have a major impact on your home life. When one member of the family has kidney cancer, the whole family has kidney cancer. The love and support of family members are important in every phase of diagnosis and treatment. When the disease is first diagnosed, the family can comfort the patient. When the patient is in the hospital, family members often supplement the nursing staff in watching over the patient. When the patient comes home from the hospital, family members care for the patient. When follow-up and treatment continue, family members support the process.

Experienced doctors and nurses know that the family is hurting, and helping the family is another way to help the patient. And just as the doctor and nurse develop a relationship with the patient, they also often develop a relationship with the patient's family. This relationship with patient and family usually starts at the time of diagnosis. Most doctors will want to brief family members along with the patient about the diagnosis and plan for the patient. It helps if this briefing takes place all at one time so family members hear exactly the same things and family members get to hear the questions of other family members.

If a nephrectomy is done, the surgeon can send word of how the operation is going to waiting family members. After the operation, the surgeon will also brief the family about the patient's condition. As the patient recovers in the hospital, family members will probably meet with the patient's doctors and nurses. This contact can provide the family with an opportunity for questions and learning.

Research has shown that a person living with cancer will only remember a limited amount of information that is given during an office visit with the doctor. This happens because the patient is trying to process a lot of new information and because people remember less when dealing with a stressful situation. To increase doctor-patient communication, you should write down questions you want to have answered before arriving for your appointment. Find a family member or friend willing to accompany you to all medical appointments. This person can take notes for you while in the doctor's office and later help you clarify information. If you choose, this person can serve as a contact to provide information to the concerned, significant people in your life. It can become exhausting for patients to disseminate information about their progress to loved ones numerous times. This approach also discourages different family members from contacting the health care team individually to be briefed on the patient's condition. It's important to have a well-thought-out plan for communicating information among loved ones.

Those who experience kidney cancer may find that family becomes one of the most important factors in their recovery. Connecting with other families who have gone through the same challenges can be very helpful. The Kidney Cancer Association maintains a chat room for patients and families at its website (www.kidneycancer.org), and other chat rooms, message boards, and support groups for families facing a cancer diagnosis are common online. You can learn more about these resources and other issues related to families in the chapter "Emotional Well-Being."

Health Insurance

Like any major illness, costs for cancer treatment can be high. If you have health insurance, such as coverage through your employer, you should read all of the information brochures and details of your policy. Become familiar with the terms of your coverage and the procedures for filing claims. If your employer is a larger company, you should meet with the company's benefits administrator and/or medical director. These people can help you. It is also a good idea to have a friend or family member help you review all your medical bills, insurance claims, payments, and reimbursements.

Health plans, including insurance, are regulated by federal and state laws, and these laws may vary. Be prepared to do your homework regarding the laws in your state.

Insurance Coverage for Clinical Trials

Clinical trials of investigational treatments (those not approved by the FDA for kidney cancer) are frequently used medical options for patients dealing with advanced kidney cancer. Often, insurance companies only reimburse for recognized standard forms of treatment. Therefore, it is important to check with your insurance company regarding their reimbursement policies before beginning a specific treatment. Many clinical trial programs will do this for you so check with your doctor first before contacting your insurance company.

If you are currently in treatment and your insurance company has rejected one of your claims, there are several things you can do. First, you can simply resubmit the claim. Often, it will be processed by a different claims reviewer who may approve it. Second, many insurance companies have formal claims appeal processes. You can appeal your claim and have it reviewed. Third, if a claim is rejected after submission, and you work for a large company, you should notify your employer's benefits administrator, corporate medical director, or union benefits representative. They may be able to make suggestions or resubmit the claim for you. Your employer is the insurance company's customer, and the insurance company wants to keep customers happy. If your employer intercedes on your behalf, the claim may be paid. A good company will take this action because it pays a lot of money for its employee health insurance program. It wants to get value in return for its premiums. Fourth, you can write to your state's insurance commissioner and send a copy of the letter to your insurance company. Insurance is a regulated industry and most states have a commission or government agent who oversees insurance companies operating within the state. Your insurance company may decide to pay your claim rather than have to respond to a commission inquiry. If your insurance company is still unresponsive, you can file a formal complaint with the insurance commission in your state. Record the date and name of the person you talk to whenever you call your insurance company.

The Kidney Cancer Association does not advocate confrontation as a tactic for resolving insurance claims. History has shown that people have offered bogus cures for cancer as well as a host of other illnesses. Some have filed false insurance claims and committed insurance fraud; others have abused their coverage. It is understandable for insurance companies to be careful with the funds of their policyholders. Prudence in paying claims holds the cost of insurance down and makes it more affordable for all patients.

You stand a better chance of being reimbursed for an experimental treatment if it has the support of your doctor and other physicians, if it is administered through a major university teaching hospital, and if prior experience with the treatment indicates that it may help you. These things reassure the insurance company that your claim is not frivolous and that the treatment is appropriate even if it is unproved. Involve your doctor and hospital treatment center if you have difficulty getting support from your insurance company. Talk with the financial counselors at the hospital where you're getting treatment – they can work with your insurance company to be sure that charges were billed correctly, that correct "codes" were used, and to clarify charges. Charges for physician visits, tests, and procedures are determined based on whether or not they are considered "standard of care" for a patient with kidney cancer. Your insurance company should cover those charges that are "standard of care." Charges for tests done specifically for "research" are typically covered by the sponsor of the clinical trial that is conducting the research. Your health care team or financial counselor can help you with treatment bills and insurance issues.

Financial counselors may also be able to assist with other needs, such as co-payment assistance and other billing issues. With the passage of new federal health care reform legislation in 2010, it is possible that insurance-coverage policies and procedures may change, making a check with your insurance company doubly important.

Medicare and Medicaid

Kidney cancer patients may qualify for treatment under Medicare and Medicaid. An easy way to learn more is to ask the social services department or admissions officer at your hospital about benefits. Your hospital will have all pertinent information on these government programs. Precise benefits may vary from state to state. You should also contact your local office of the U.S. Department of Health and Human Services (HHS) or visit the Medicare website at www.medicare.gov for more information and to obtain one of the following U.S. government publications covering Medicare:

"Medicare & You."
Contains detailed facts about Medicare benefits and the health plan options available to you. Publication number 10050.

"Medicare and Home Health Care."
This pamphlet provides information about home health care under Medicare. Publication number 10969.

"Medicare Hospice Benefits."
Hospice care is a special type of care for terminally ill patients. Learn how to find hospice programs and where to get information. Publication number 02154.

"Medicare Preventive Services"
Use this guide to lower your risk of cancer, flu, pneumonia, diabetes, etc. Publication number 10110.

"Where to Get Your Medicare Questions Answered."
This guide provides the latest information in an easy-to-understand question-and-answer format, including definitions of important terms. Publication number 02246.

"Your Medicare Benefits."
This pamphlet provides information about what your health care plan covers.

You can also obtain these publications by calling toll-free 1-888-878-3256, by writing to the Federal Citizen Information Center, Department WWW, Pueblo, CO 81009, or by visiting their website at http://www.pueblo.gsa.gov.

For specific questions about the Medicaid program, visit www.cms.hhs.gov/home/medicaid.asp.

Social Security Disability Benefits

The Social Security Administration (SSA) is the government agency that oversees Social Security and Supplemental Security Income (SSI). Some cancer patients may receive a monthly income from the Social Security Administration (SSA) if they meet its disability standards.

Benefits from SSA are available to cancer patients who have worked and paid social security taxes and now are considered disabled: That is, they cannot do work they did before, and their disability is expected to last for at least one year or to result in death.

In determining your disability, the SSA will consider a range of factors. You can learn more about the process and whether you might be eligible for benefits by visiting the SSA website at www.ssa.gov or by calling 800-772-1213.

Life Insurance

It may seem strange to think about getting or increasing your life insurance coverage after you have cancer. However, there are many reasons you may need to obtain or increase your life insurance. For example, if you seek to borrow money or want a home mortgage, your bank may require that a life insurance policy be in force, naming the bank as the beneficiary. If you own a business or have business partners, your company may need to carry a life insurance policy on you to buy back your stock in the event of death.

Increasing numbers of cancer patients survive their disease. The longer you survive, the more likely you are cured, and the better you are viewed as an acceptable risk by the insurance companies. There are insurance companies willing to provide coverage to cancer patients if they no longer show disease and a suitable amount of time has passed since the initial treatment and diagnosis.

If you wish to obtain life insurance or increase your coverage, talk with a qualified insurance agent to explore what might be available. Be aware that you may be assigned to a high-risk class and pay a higher price for coverage than someone who has not had cancer.

Employment and Business

Your employer will probably learn that you have kidney cancer because you will be missing from work for several weeks while you have a nephrectomy. You may also miss work if you participate in certain clinical trials or treatments. Also, your insurance claim submissions may have to be signed by your employer.

Your relationship to your job is a very important factor in your quality of life. If you are unhappy in your job, your cancer may serve as motivation for you to think about changing jobs. If you have a high-stress job or one that demands a lot of extra time or extensive travel, you may want to switch jobs within the same organization.

Even though you may be cured of cancer, an employer may perceive you as a risky employee or an employee who is going to be more expensive to insure or who is going to require time off. Nevertheless, laws are in place to protect you against discrimination. The Americans with Disabilities Act is a Federal law which prevents job discrimination against people with a cancer history. ERISA is Federal law which governs employer health benefits. The Medicare and Medicaid programs are also governed by Federal laws.

Your health condition will also be a factor if you are searching for a new job. Most employers have a policy of giving job candidates pre-employment physicals. Your health record will also be part of any employer insurance application, and your employer may have to sign these forms when they are submitted to the insurance company for approval.

Employment Discrimination

If you are denied a job because of your cancer, you may consider filing a complaint with the federal government. Under the

Rehabilitation Act of 1973, any U.S. government contractor or subcontractor receiving $50,000 or more, and with 50 or more employees, is required to prepare and maintain an affirmative action program for the handicapped. Moreover, employers that receive any money from the Department of Health and Human Services are required to maintain such a program regardless of size or amount of money received.

Cancer patients are classified as handicapped under this law. If you suffer job discrimination because of your cancer, you can file a complaint under Section 503 of the Rehabilitation Act with the Office of Federal Contract Compliance Programs of the U.S. Department of Labor. If your complaint involves a contractor for the Department of Health and Human Services, it will fall under Section 504 of the law and should be filed with the Office of Civil Rights at the Department of Health and Human Services. Your state Department of Labor or Office of Civil Rights may also be responsible for enforcing state laws prohibiting discrimination against people with a cancer history. Many states have enacted statutes designed to protect those deemed disabled.

The Cancer Legal Resource Center (CLRC) is a joint program of the Disability Rights Legal Center and Loyola Law School. The CLRC provides a variety of free resources on cancer-related legal issues to cancer survivors, caregivers, health care professionals and others. Visit www.disabilityrightslegalcenter.org to learn more about these resources.

Employment Benefits

On the plus side, because you have been recognized as handicapped by the federal government under the Rehabilitation Act of 1973, an employer may be eligible for federal and state job credits, training grants, and other forms of financial assistance as a result of your employment. To find out more, contact your state Department of Labor before you seek a new job.

If you own a company that does business with the federal, state, or city government, it may be eligible for preferential treatment in contract bidding. Companies that are federal contractors or subcontractors may also give preferential treatment to suppliers owned by handicapped persons because it helps them fulfill obligations under federal statutes. It may seem strange to profit from having cancer, but you didn't decide to get cancer and you didn't write the laws pertaining to handicapped persons.

The Impact of Laws on Cancer Patients

Laws are the formal rules that run a society. Many federal and state laws affect you as a cancer patient. The U.S. Food and Drug Administration is empowered and governed by laws passed by Congress. The budget for the National Cancer Institute is set each year by an appropriations law passed by Congress.

These laws influence the quality and availability of your health care, what you pay for your care, and many other aspects of your care. It is important for you to know your rights and restrictions under various laws.

The Kidney Cancer Association tracks important legal developments that relate to patient rights and patient care. The Association also educates members of Congress, government agencies, and other organizations about the needs of kidney cancer patients. For example, the Association has organized meetings between patients and members of Congress. The Association has also testified before Congressional hearings on the needs of patients. To learn more about the Association's work related to patients' rights and patient care, visit www.kidneycancer.org.

Reach Out to Others for Support

"I was diagnosed with a tumor in my right kidney. Two other doctors looked at the scans and didn't see anything else, but a fourth doctor detected another tumor in my left kidney. I had bilateral tumors, which are rare. After the bilateral diagnosis I was in shock, but remained hopeful until my third and most invasive surgery, an open partial nephrectomy with rib removal, three years later. After that I became very depressed.

I had just about given up hope when a notice arrived in the mail about an upcoming kidney cancer conference. My husband saw the announcement and he suggested we go, but I resisted. With a push from him, I said "OK, I'll go." Up until then I felt all alone with my disease, but when I got to the conference I connected with a lot of other people with kidney cancer and I started to feel better. The information at the conference was great and I started thinking that maybe I should share it with others. The Kidney Cancer Association encouraged me to go to some other conferences and that led to me becoming a host for meetings of kidney cancer patients in my local area. At the first meeting we had 30 people or more and the room was packed.

Now we get together three or four times a year, often bringing in a doctor to speak. We exchange new information that we gather from conferences, or from studies and research. What are the new treatments? Any new developments in surgery? And so on. The meetings are very educational – we are there to exchange information, not feel sorry for ourselves. It only takes an hour or so for the meeting. We have some refreshments, and then everything kind of flows along.

The interaction between the other patients is awesome. I've formed new friendships as a result – we meet for lunch and coffee and generally support each other. I would strongly encourage others to consider organizing a meeting in your local area. The first step is to call the Kidney Cancer Association, which will provide advice and assistance in getting started. Becoming involved this way has been a huge boost for me. I continue to meet with others because I know a lot of people feel isolated, like I was. When they come to the meeting I know I've helped somebody – and they usually walk away with a sense that there's hope."

CHAPTER 10

EMOTIONAL WELL-BEING

Good mental health goes hand-in-hand with good physical health.
Your state of mind is an important part of fighting kidney cancer.

Mental Health

As you experience cancer, you will encounter books and articles advocating a positive mental attitude, intimate and loving relationships, reduction of stress, imaging, meditation, and other relaxation techniques. The real message of these writings is that mental processes and states of mind can contribute to survival and healing in cancer patients. In short, good mental health goes hand-in-hand with good physical health. A positive mental attitude is free. It does not require a doctor or a hospital or an insurance company.

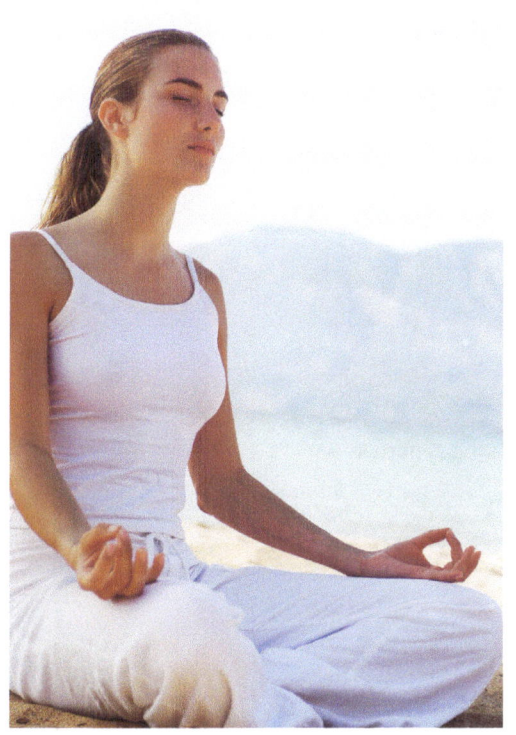

Good mental health goes hand in hand with good physical health. Pay attention to your emotional well being.

There is a body of research on how psychological processes and the central nervous system interact with the immune system. Thought processes involve chemical communications among neurons in the brain and central nervous system. The immune system also communicates chemically with the central nervous system to perform a variety of functions.

Research indicates that stress can alter immune system function. In turn, immune system function can alter tumor growth and response. Disease and treatment are stressful, and this stress may also alter immune function. Stress reduction, imaging, and visualization techniques are thought to be useful in cancer treatment because of this linkage.

Cancer Wellness

Cancer wellness is the promotion of health and general well-being in people with cancer and those close to them. Wellness operates at four levels: physical, functional, emotional, and social.

The physical condition of cancer dominates the other three levels. If you didn't have a tumor and the disease, cancer wellness would not be an issue. The physical aspect of cancer presents itself with symptoms and possible side effects from treatment. Your physical condition can limit your ability to function normally in your work, recreation, and daily life. Your performance, from sleeping to household chores, may be affected.

If functional performance is lessened, emotional distress, frustration, and loss of well-being may result. The spiritual side of your life may be affected and personality change may result. Sociability, intimacy, and family functioning may also be diminished. Stressful family conflicts may result as tension increases within the family. These are symptoms of emotional and social discomfort, and can be eliminated or diminished through counseling.

Cancer patients typically experience three types of psychological difficulty: the "Damocles Syndrome," which refers to uncertainty about one's health and the fear that cancer may return; the "Lazarus Syndrome," which refers to the difficulty patients have being treated normally as they re-enter the healthy, productive world; and the "Residual Stress Syndrome," which refers to the anxiety that comes from having had cancer. These are normal consequences of having cancer. In part, just as you may have a physical scar from surgery, you have a "mental scar" from your cancer experience.

If you or your family has unusual distress from an encounter with kidney cancer, you may wish to seek professional counseling. These services may be covered by your insurance. Your doctor can refer you to a mental health professional. Many cancer centers have psychologists and social workers that specialize in assisting cancer patients and their families. It may be helpful for you to take advantage of these services. Many patients and families do and benefit from the experience.

Helping Yourself

David F. Cella, PhD, a clinical psychologist who works with cancer patients, has developed a cancer wellness doctrine consisting of eight commonly held beliefs, plus eight modifiers. As you seek cancer wellness, you should keep these eight modifiers in mind:

My health is my responsibility. (But I did not cause my disease.) Take charge, but don't blame yourself. No one really knows what causes a particular case of kidney cancer.

I will always have hope. (But what I hope for may change over time.) Goals and aspirations change throughout life, even if you don't have cancer.

My doctor and I are partners. (We both have things to learn.) Be open to new ideas and be actively involved in your treatment.

Death is not failure. (Personal dignity and quality of life are my measures of success.) Work to make your life better.

Cancer provides me with an opportunity. (But I don't have to be grateful for it, and I didn't need it.) It's okay to dislike the cancer experience, but it pays to make the best of it.

I can change the way I deal with stress. (The past is unimportant unless I make it so.) Avoid excessive stress and look forward to future pleasures and experiences.

Cancer is a family illness. (Therefore, my family needs attention too.) Don't take your family relationships for granted. Build new dimensions into your relationships.

I can make a difference in my care. (I need to look inside myself for the proper direction.) You really do know the right thing for you to do. Proceed thoughtfully and trust yourself.

Support Groups

Support groups can also be beneficial in reducing the anxiety levels of cancer patients and their caregivers. Patients and family members can attend groups together or join separate groups designed to meet their specific needs. Newly diagnosed patients and their supporters frequently obtain useful information and receive emotional support by talking to a cancer survivor who has undergone a similar type of treatment and can share his or her experiences. The emotional benefits these groups can provide are significant. Support groups have greatly improved the quality of life of many people who have been diagnosed with cancer.

A person living with kidney cancer needs to be selective in choosing a group. Because the cancer is rare and recommended treatments are often different from those for other cancers, the kidney cancer patient may have difficulty obtaining needed information from other cancer survivors or relating to them. To accommodate the special needs of the kidney cancer patient, the Kidney Cancer Association conducts patient meetings at major cities throughout the country. In addition, the Association's regional patient conferences are a good place to meet many other kidney cancer survivors and their families and learn about new treatments and clinical trials. To obtain more immediate information, you may call the Association (1-800-850-9132) and ask to talk to another survivor or family member who has volunteered to be a resource for you.

Talking With Children About Cancer and Treatment

While this can be a very difficult topic, it's important to be honest and up-front with children about cancer. Bringing children to an appointment so they can see "how things work" and meet the medical team can be very helpful as they try to understand your cancer diagnosis. By bringing children along on a medical visit, they will have the chance to share their feelings and ask questions. It may be necessary to take children out of school for the day, but the result can be positive, helping them feel they are a part of things, rather than being left out. It also helps you and other family members remember to deal with the needs of children throughout the diagnosis and treatment process. Being referred to a Child-Life Specialist, if available, can be helpful for you and your children. Ask your oncology provider if one is in your area.

Finding Support Online

If you have a computer and access to the Internet, you may also participate in online support groups, such as message boards, chat rooms or reading individual blogs. An online message board allows individual participants to communicate with a group of people who share ideas and questions. New messages are posted throughout the day. The Kidney Cancer Association offers a message board where patients can share information on its website.

Chat rooms are also a useful online tool, allowing participants to meet online in real time. The Kidney Cancer Association's chat room gives participants the opportunity to see messages as they are being typed, enabling participants to "talk" with one another. The chat room is always open and one group meets weekly. To learn more about the Kidney Cancer Association's message board or chat room, visit www.kidneycancer.org.

Individual blogs can also be helpful, because they may give the personal experiences of an individual with kidney cancer. However, it is important to understand that each person with kidney cancer will experience kidney cancer differently and what happens in one case may not reflect what happens in another.

The Kidney Cancer Association also offers a live support feature that enables website visitors to directly contact the Association office and be put in touch with people who are knowledgeable about the treatment of kidney cancer. This service is available during office hours, Monday through Friday. You can also contact the Association office by calling 1-800-850-9132.

It is important to understand that not everything on the Internet comes from a reliable source. Consider carefully the credibility of the website before you draw any conclusions. The resources chapter of this book offers a number of reliable websites.

Palliative Care

Palliative care (or supportive care) is a specialty that focuses on comfort and improving quality of life for patients of any age with serious illness such as cancer. Palliative care is not intended to treat or cure the cancer itself, but to be an additional resource to you for optimizing your quality of life, while you are receiving treatment. Palliative care providers help with treating symptoms, pain, and stress caused by the cancer or treatment. It is provided to support the patient and family during treatment. Many cancer treatment centers have dedicated palliative care doctors and nurses and other specialists who can give additional support in helping patients and their families in meeting their treatment goals.

Oncology doctors and nurses can also deliver palliative care if a palliative care team is not available. Palliative care can help throughout the cancer journey and is an important part of cancer treatment. It not only can help with symptoms such as nausea, pain, fatigue and shortness of breath but also can help a patient deal with emotional and spiritual issues. Palliative care supports patients by having them take part in decisions about care and assuring that all care needs are met. Studies have shown that people who participate in palliative care support have a better quality of life, less severe symptoms, and may also have an increase in survival. Discuss palliative care with your doctor so he or she can address your needs. Great strides have been made in recent years in developing palliative care options. Palliative care services exist in both inpatient and outpatient settings, and much of the actual care can be done at home.

Hospice Care

It is perfectly normal for someone with kidney cancer to think about the possibility of dying of the disease. Denying that you have cancer or denying the possibility of death is not okay. Denial of this possibility is likely to cause you more problems and stress than squarely facing it. You may not like your situation, but at least you should attempt to understand it and improve on it. You should not give up living just because you have cancer. Enjoy life and savor every moment. Set new goals and work to achieve them. Don't make your cancer and the possibility of death the sole driving force in your life.

At some point in your illness the decision may be made to transition to care that focuses on quality of life and comfort care rather than further anti-cancer treatment. This is a decision made by you in collaboration with your physician and family. The focus of Hospice and "End of Life care" is to control symptoms, with an emphasis on psychological, spiritual, and social support for patients and families facing terminal illness. Hospice helps you make the most of your remaining time, with an emphasis on quality rather than quantity.

Hospice care is care that focuses on giving medical, psychological, and spiritual support and its goal is to give people who are dying peace, comfort, and dignity. It provides compassionate care for people in the last stages of incurable diseases, such as cancer, so that they may have optimal quality of life and be as comfortable as possible. Being enrolled in hospice does not mean you are "giving up" or that hope is gone. If you get better, or the cancer goes into remission, you can leave hospice. Hospice brings the hope of quality of life and optimizing each day.

Hospice philosophy accepts death as the final stage of life and treats the person rather than the disease. The patient and family are included in making decisions.

Life is precious. However, one cannot truly celebrate life without also thinking about death. Death is a natural part of life and we will all share the experience. From the moment we enter the world, it is certain that we will leave it. What counts is the trip along the way.

Be sure to communicate your end of life concerns to your doctor and family. For example, you may want to decide whether you want to stay in the hospital or spend your remaining time at home. Avoid hospitalization when the goal of your treatment is comfort measures. Ask your doctor or hospital or clinic social worker about a hospice program, or contact the National Hospice and Palliative Care Organization, 1731 King Street, Suite 100, Alexandria, VA 22314; telephone 1-703-837-1500; website: www.nhpco.org.

Make time for yourself and seek spiritual counsel if doing so would help you. An important thing to consider is spending special time with each of your loved ones. This special time can create lasting memories for them.

Life and death are unique and personal experiences. None of us will have exactly the same experience as another person. No one can live for us. No one can die for us. We achieve success when we have peace of mind – when we are comfortable with ourselves and in harmony with the world around us.

If you would like more guidance on these issues, the Kidney Cancer Association offers a book, "Reflections: A Guide to End of Life Issues," written by Roger C. Bone, MD, a doctor and kidney cancer patient. The book may be downloaded at www.kidneycancer.org.

Legal Matters

As a practical matter, if you don't have a will, this is an appropriate time to make one. If you already have one, review it with an attorney. If you don't have an attorney, call the local chapter of the American Bar Association or your state bar association for assistance or contact your Legal Aid Society.

The U.S. Supreme Court has recognized your constitutional right to refuse medical care, including life support, even when such a refusal results in death. However, your right to die may be subject to state laws requiring evidence of your personal wishes and desires. Two types of legal documents can be used to express your wishes: the Healthcare Power of Attorney, also known more commonly as the "advance directive," and the Living Will.

A Healthcare Power of Attorney is a broad document that delegates decision-making authority over your health care to another individual, usually a spouse or other close relative. The Healthcare Power of Attorney enables your designated agent to authorize hospitalization, personal care, and medical treatment, as well as to withhold or withdraw any medical treatment. For example, the Healthcare Power of Attorney can permit your agent to withdraw food and water or life support systems under certain conditions according to your wishes. It is helpful for the medical team to have a designated person with whom they can discuss specific issues if you are unable to do so as a result of your medical condition.

A Living Will is a simple document that gives instructions to your doctor and family about your desires should you become incapacitated and cannot express them at a later time. Through your Living Will, you can give instructions to your doctor and family about how you want to be treated while you are alive but unable to speak for yourself. For example, you may instruct your doctor to withdraw death-delaying treatment if you are in a "terminal" condition and death is imminent.

Seek the counsel of a professional estate-planning attorney in drafting the necessary documents. By expressing your wishes clearly and forcefully, you can relieve your family and loved ones of very difficult decisions regarding your care. They will not wonder whether they have made correct decisions and they will have no anxiety or guilt. They will simply carry out your wishes as you specify them.

The Importance of Hope – and Positive Emotions

A kidney cancer diagnosis may be traumatic to both you and your family. Remember, though, that there is hope – new drugs and treatments are advancing rapidly, and the prognosis for kidney cancer patients is better today than it was just a few years ago. After your diagnosis, you will be presented with many tools to help in your recovery, ranging from surgery to therapeutic care. Among those tools, one of the most important is your own state of mind – don't underestimate its power in bringing you back to good health.

NOTES

Choose the right doctor and build a positive mental attitude

Patient: Keith
Age: 63

"I was diagnosed with kidney cancer on a Saturday and had a nephrectomy on the following Wednesday. That's how dire my situation was. So I didn't have much time to research the disease. We had to act quickly.

My symptom was muscle pain in my shoulder. I thought I had hurt myself working out, and the initial treatment from my doctor was to take an anti-inflammatory. But when the pain persisted, an MRI showed that I had a growth on my spine. My kidney cancer had metastasized to a cervical vertebra. I had to have a laminectomy on my vertebra, then IL2.

Afterwards, I learned a great deal, mostly by spending a lot of time seeking out information online. There is a wealth of information on the Internet. This was important as I prepared for IL2 therapy. Since I completed my IL2 treatment, I've been living a normal life. I've had to make some adjustments, mostly related to the laminectomy, but overall things are good.

My advice to other kidney cancer patients would be first of all, to make sure you get the right oncologist. Interview three or four if you have to. Find someone who really specializes in your disease. Seek out the best you can find.

If you have to go through IL2, or any other adjuvant therapy, take the time to work on building a positive outlook. I used positive-visioning exercises during my therapy, and there are numerous other ways to work on your mental and emotional state, which is vital for your recovery. This shouldn't be underestimated. You need both a positive mental attitude and the therapy itself. The two work together." And of course, it helped that I had a wonderful and supportive wife. Strong family support can be an important ingredient in recovery."

CHAPTER 11

RESOURCES FOR PATIENTS AND FAMILIES

Learn more and get connected – you may be able to help someone else in addition to yourself.

This book provides essential background to help you understand the basics of a kidney cancer diagnosis. But much more detailed information is available from a variety of other sources. Use this chapter to add to your knowledge.

Cancer Organizations

Kidney Cancer Association

Publications*, patient meetings, support groups, educational meetings, medication information sheets, webinars, patient conferences, online support, videos, e-newsletter: Kidney Cancer News.

> Call 1-800-850-9132.
> www.kidneycancer.org,
> E-mail: office@kidneycancer.org

*May have publications in several languages.

National Cancer Institute

> Call 1-800-4-CANCER (1-800-422-6237).
> http://cis.nci.nih.gov
> Kidney Cancer: http://web.ncifcrf.gov/research/kidney
> Clinical Trials: http://cancertrials.nci.nih.gov

American Cancer Society

Educational programs and support group information through network of local offices. Materials include booklets, videos, and audiotapes; many also available in Spanish.

> Call 1-800-ACS-2345.
> www.cancer.org

National Comprehensive Cancer Network

Patient and care giver information and resources. Also patient and disease guidelines for treatment.

> www. nccn.org

Society of Immunotherapy of Cancer (SITC)

SITC has relationships with government, regulatory agencies, patient advocacy organizations and foundations.

http://kidneycancertrials.com

Cancer Centers

Cancer Information Offices are part of many hospitals, particularly those that are **Comprehensive Cancer Centers**. These centers specialize in research and treatment and are recognized by the **National Cancer Institute**.

For the name, address, and phone number of the nearest center, call the **Cancer Information Service** at 1-800-4-CANCER.

Clinical Trials Information

See these websites for up to date information on clinical trials.

National Cancer Institute

www.cancer.gov/clinicaltrials

National Institute of Health

www.clinicaltrials.gov

Complementary and Alternative Medicine (CAM)

National Center for Complementary and Alternative Medicine

http://nccam.nih.gov

Drug Treatment/Patient Information

Patient Resources

www.kidneycancer.org.

Afinitor® (everolimus)

www.afinitor.com/index.jsp

Avastin® (bevacizumab)

www.avastin.com

Cabometyx® (cabozantinib)

https://hcp.cabometyx.com

Inlyta® (axitinib)

www.inlyta.com

Intron A® (interferon)

www.merck.com/product/oncology/home.html

Lenvima® (lenvantinib)
    www.lenvima.com

Nexavar® (sorafenib)
    www.nexavar.com

Opdivo® (nivolumab)
    www.opdivotherapy.com

Proleukin® (interleukin-2)
    www.proleukin.com

Sutent® (sunitinib)
    www.sutent.com

Torisel® (temsirolimus)
    www.torisel.com

Votrient® (pazopanib)
    www.us.votrient.com

Emotional Support Resources

Cancercare
    www.cancercare.org

Cancer Net (ASCO site for patients & families)
    www.cancer.net/Cancer/cancer.html

4th Angel Mentoring Program
www.clevelandclinic.org/cancer/scottcares/4thangel/about.asp

ChemoCare.com
    www.chemocare.com

Educational Resources

Anti-angiogensis website
    www.newfrontierincancer.org

International Kidney Cancer Symposia

The Kidney Cancer Association hosts the International Kidney Cancer Symposium and the European International Kidney Cancer Symposium. These meetings, for urologists, oncologists, researchers, nurses and other health care professionals, provide a forum for learning about what's new in the area of kidney cancer as well as new treatment agents. Full proceedings of the International Kidney Cancer Symposium, including video presentations and slide shows, are available at
    www.kidneycancer.org.

The Kidney Cancer Journal

www.kidneycancerjournal.org

Patient Centered Guides

www.patientcenters.com

Support for Disability Assistance

Social Security Administration

www.ssa.gov
Telephone: 800-772-1213

Disability Rights Legal Center

www.disabilityrightslegalcenter.org

GLOSSARY OF TERMS

Ablation: The surgical removal of body tissue.

Adjuvant Treatment: An additional treatment designed to help reach the ultimate therapeutic goal. Adjuvant therapy for cancer may refer to surgery followed by chemotherapy, for example.

Angiogenesis Inhibitors: Unique cancer-fighting agents that tend to inhibit the growth of blood vessels rather than tumor cells. In some cancers, angiogenesis inhibitors are most effective when combined with additional therapies, especially chemotherapy.

Arterial Embolization: A procedure where a catheter is used to deliver small particles that block the blood supply to a tumor.

Biopsy: An examination of tissue removed from a living body to discover the presence, cause, or extent of a disease.

Bone Marrow Transplant: Also called a stem cell transplant, Bone Marrow Transplant is a procedure that infuses healthy cells, called stem cells, into the body to replace damaged or diseased bone marrow. A bone marrow transplant may also be used to treat certain types of cancer.

Cancer Staging: The process of determining how much cancer is in the body and where it is located. Staging describes the severity of an individual's cancer based on the magnitude of the original (primary) tumor as well as on the extent cancer has spread in the body.

Chemotherapy: A form of therapy that uses anti-cancer (cytotoxic) drugs to destroy cancer cells. The drugs also affect healthy cells, causing side effects such as feeling sick or an increased risk of infection. Unlike cancer cells, these healthy cells usually repair themselves.

Chromophobe Renal Cell Carcinoma: A rare type of kidney cancer, representing 5% of cases. There is a familial or inherited form of Chromophobe RCC called Birth-Hogg-Dub Syndrome, which is also associated with a specific genetic syndrome.

Clinical Trials: Research studies that explore whether a medical strategy, treatment, or device is safe and effective for humans. These studies also may show which medical approaches work best for certain illnesses or groups of people.

Collecting Duct Carcinoma (CDC): Also known as Bellini duct carcinoma, CDC is a type of kidney cancer that originates in the papillary duct of the kidney.

Complementary and Alternative Medicine (CAM): A category of medicine that includes a variety of treatment approaches that fall outside the realm of conventional medicine.

Computerized Tomography (CT) Scan: A medical imaging process that combines a series of X-ray images taken from different angles and uses a computer to create cross-sectional images of the bones, blood vessels and soft tissues inside the body.

Healthcare Power of Attorney: A legal directive that authorizes someone to act as an individual's formally recognized agent and on their behalf in healthcare decision-making.

Hospice Care: A specialized care designed to provide support to patients and families during an advanced illness. Hospice care focuses on comfort and quality of life, rather than cure.

Immunotherapy: Also known as biologic therapy, Immunotherapy is a type of cancer treatment designed to boost the body's natural defenses to fight the cancer. It uses substances either made by the body or in a laboratory to improve or restore immune system function.

Interferons: A family of naturally-occurring proteins that are made and secreted by cells of the immune system (for example, white blood cells). They have been widely used to treat cancer, alone or in combination with other drugs.

Interleukin-2: A chemical substance used in the treatment of advanced kidney cancer. It stimulates the growth of white blood cells.

Laparoscopy: A surgical procedure in which a fiber-optic instrument is inserted through the abdominal wall to view the organs in the abdomen or to permit a surgical procedure.

Living Will: A written statement detailing an individual's desires regarding their medical treatment in circumstances in which they are no longer able to express informed consent.

Lymph Nodes: Small, bean-shaped glands throughout the body. They are part of the lymph system, which carries fluid (lymph fluid), nutrients, and waste material between the body tissues and the bloodstream.

Magnetic Resonance Imaging: A form of medical imaging that measures the response of body tissues to high-frequency radio waves when placed in a strong magnetic field, producing images of the internal organs.

Mammalian Target of Rapamycin (mTOR):
A serine/threonine kinase, which belongs to phosphatidylinositol-3 kinase (PI3K) related kinases (PIKKs) family and regulates cellular metabolism, growth, and proliferation. Because of its role in cell growth, it is a target for the development of mTOR inhibitors – chemical agents that are used to fight kidney cancer tumors.

Monoclonal Antibodies: Proteins produced by the body's immune system that fight infections and foreign substances in the body.

Nephrectomy: The surgical removal of one or both of the kidneys.

Palliative Care: A specialty that focuses on comfort and improving quality of life for patients of any age with a serious illness, such as cancer. Palliative care is not intended to treat or cure the cancer itself, but is an additional resource for optimizing the patient's quality of life while receiving treatment.

Papillary Renal Cell Carcinoma (PRCC): The second most common type of kidney cancer, which forms inside the lining of the kidney's tubules. There is an increased incidence of PRCC in African Americans.

Positron Emission Tomography (PET) Scan: A medical imaging process that uses a special dye injected into the arm to make the organs and tissues of the body viewable.

Radiation Therapy: One of the most common treatments for cancer, using high-energy particles or waves, such as x-rays, gamma rays, electron beams, or protons, to destroy or damage cancer cells.

Renal Cell Carcinoma (RCC): A disease in which malignant cancer cells are found in the lining of tubules (very small tubes) in the kidney. It is the most common type of kidney cancer in adults.

Renal Medullary Carcinoma: A rare type of cancer that affects the kidney. It tends to be aggressive, difficult to treat, and is often metastatic at the time of diagnosis.

Renal Oncocytoma: A tumor of the kidney made up of oncocytes, a special kind of cell.

Sarcomatoid RCC: A variant of kidney cancer that results in aggressive tumors that respond poorly to some therapies. The condition is found frequently in patients whose kidney cancer has metastasized widely.

Targeted Therapy: A newer type of cancer treatment that uses drugs or other substances to more precisely identify and attack cancer cells, usually while doing little damage to normal cells. Targeted therapy is a growing part of many cancer treatment regimens.

Transitional Cell Carcinoma of the Kidney: A rare and potentially very aggressive tumor that is not considered a true kidney cancer, but instead is grouped with bladder cancer.

Ultrasound Scan: A medical test that uses high-frequency sound waves to capture live images from the inside of the body. It's also known as sonography.

Unclassified RCC: A heterogeneous group of tumors not fitting into other kidney cancer subtypes, with a highly variable clinical course.

Vaccine Therapy: A type of treatment that uses a substance or group of substances to stimulate the immune system to destroy a tumor or infectious microorganisms, such as bacteria or viruses.

About The Kidney Cancer Association

In 1989, a group of kidney cancer patients started to meet and discuss their experiences and the lack of information available about their disease. Out of these meetings, the Kidney Cancer Association was formed and officially incorporated as a non-profit organization in March of 1990.

The Association has three basic purposes. First, it provides information to patients and physicians. This book is one example. The Association can also provide you with other information through regional patient meetings and via its website, which is located at www.kidneycancer.org. Second, the Association sponsors research on kidney cancer and encourages others to conduct research on the disease. Only a small percentage of all cancer cases are kidney cancers. Compared to other, more common cancers, little research is done on kidney cancer. Third, the Association acts as an advocate on behalf of kidney cancer patients and their families. The Association speaks at public hearings to support policies that will improve the care and treatment of cancer patients.

How You Can Join

Patients, families, physicians, nurses, other healthcare professionals, corporations, and the public at large can join the Kidney Cancer Association by calling the headquarters office at 1-800-850-9132 or by sending an email to office@kidneycancer.org.

Just leave your name, address, telephone number and email address. You can also become a member by visiting the website at www.kidneycancer.org and clicking on "Login." You will be added to the Association's mailing list and you will receive *Kidney Cancer News*, the Association's e-newsletter. You will also receive announcements about meetings and other activities of the Association.

To achieve its purpose, the Kidney Cancer Association requests donations from members and other organizations (corporate sponsors). If you cannot afford to make a minimal donation, you can still join the Association. No one is turned away. However, the services and research sponsored by the Association cost money, so please be generous. It's the only way we can meet patient needs.

The Association also receives memorial and honorary donations made by friends on behalf of deceased kidney cancer patients. You may wish, for example, to include the Kidney Cancer Association in your will as a beneficiary. If you are interested in these forms of giving, please call us.

Your involvement in the Kidney Cancer Association will benefit you, your family, and kidney cancer patients. Act in your own self-interest and in the interest of others. Join today!

Special Note for Physicians

Physicians are especially welcome as members of the Association. The Association sponsors annual International Symposia for physicians, and it offers research grants to physicians and scientists. The Association is guided by a Medical Advisory Board of leading oncologists and urologists who are available for consultation.